GE-NOSTIC
MAN

"While working in Hollywood for over 25 years, with some of the biggest names in the business, I've seen the toll hard work and stress can have on a man. The mental and physical lifestyle adjustments listed in Michael's book will put any man back on their top game. On the job and in the bedroom!"
Matthew Booth, Hollywood film editor/director

"From my early days of growing up with my family's success with the James Bond productions, I have seen some 007 agents age better than others, and this always left an impression on me as I myself started to age. This humorous autobiography by Michael Hogg reveals how some men make terrific findings in real health solutions. I highly recommend it"
Tony Broccoli, Hollywood film producer

"Josiah Wedgwood, a master of chemistry, used his science and business skills to push the boundaries of innovation to improve and enhance people's lives. It is great to see this same spirit in Michael Hogg and so beautifully articulated in his book. The solution to achieving a better and longer tomorrow exists today. A read that fundamentally changed the way I live, yet are principles my eighth generation grandfather lived by."
Thomas Wedgwood, direct descendant of Josiah Wedgwood, founder of renowned pottery company

"Now I see ageing with men in a new way. If ageing has always baffled you, this book is the key to changing your perspective on life despite the strong influence of culture and customs. Michael, through his journey as an age-nostic man, will help you identify and connect the dots to pursue a new dream. I truly believe that women can also benefit from the age-nostic lifestyle in many ways. Thanks, Michael, for revealing your secrets to men on how to reverse the clock."
Ghada Al Rashid, brand founder and owner

"Michael's story is truly fascinating! As a producer I read a lot of interesting stories but I have never read a book that made men such fun to analyze and understand."
Julia Verdin, film producer

THE AGE-NOSTIC MAN

The secrets of anti-ageing for men

MICHAEL HOGG

Contributions from
Dr. Michael Zacharia
Tim Watson-Munro

LONDON MADRID
NEW YORK MEXICO CITY
BOGOTA BUENOS AIRES
BARCELONA MONTERREY

Published by
LID Publishing Ltd.
6-8 Underwood Street
London N1 7JQ (United Kingdom)
info@lidpublishing.com
LIDPUBLISHING.COM

A member of:

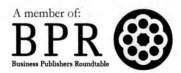

BPR
Business Publishers Roundtable

www.businesspublishersroundtable.com

Printed In Great Britain by TJInternational Ltd, Padstow, Cornwall.

ISBN: 978-1-907794-34-6

This book contains details of products and treatments that the
author has used which he believes has greatly improved his
health and well-being. Please note, however, that the information
contained within this book does not constitute medical advice
and does not amount to a general endorsement of any product.
Anyone looking to undergo treatment of a similar kind should
consult their doctor.

CONTENTS

CONTENTS

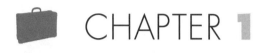

CHAPTER 1

INTRODUCTION

"Age-nostic" – What's that all about?

What is the age-nostic approach to life and why write a book about it? First, you won't find this term in any dictionary, as the word "age-nostic" does not exist in the English language. I hope it will one day, as a small yet significant vindication of this emerging field. It was 2am one morning when I woke up trying to think of a term to describe this new frontier. It came to me like a flash. "Age-nostic" seemed to me to describe a new way of life for men over 40 years of age. It encapsulates my belief that the way we have perceived and understood ageing in the past is no longer relevant.

I have searched long and hard but have not come across anyone who has delved into the immense array of anti-ageing choices, medicines, supplements and treatments that are available right now with the same passion as me. There are numerous books if you really go searching, but nothing that puts everything into one place and certainly nothing specifically tailored toward the lost tribe of the emasculated men of today. No one I have ever met truly looks forward to ageing. This book is unashamedly written for men, because we have been the ones who have been left behind to date from a medical and research perspective.

The age-nostic lifestyle is a new way to live and a better way to live. More importantly, it is a vastly better way to enjoy the second part of our life than what is presently on offer. After researching, testing and quite frankly becoming a human guinea pig, I have felt the incredible results and the changes that the age-nostic lifestyle has given me. I believe they are profoundly life changing and hugely positive. The lifestyle encompasses what my colleagues and I call the three pillars of age-nostic medicine. These are *mood, energy* and *vitality*. We believe the three pillars are the core elements of living a full and happy life for as long as we can. It is about getting back to looking great, feeling great and enjoying life in a way we

9

didn't believe possible. Or, if you choose to start early enough, it is about arresting the years and retaining a youthful body and mind for much longer than you ever expected.

These are the essential components of living a great life and when one of them – or worse still, all of them – begin to fade, life can lose its appeal and sparkle. These pillars keep us excited and positive, and they are the things that the ageing process erodes over time. They are all interconnected and work in unison. If we are depressed, have a lack of energy, or if our sex life has declined to a degree where we no longer get enjoyment from it, then all the success, money and material wealth we have accumulated will mean very little. If we can get the three pillars working again, life can be richly enjoyable and the compound effect is profound. Many people that I know have also drawn strength from the fact that they have cheated the process. We can start feeling better, looking better and in many cases take back 10 to 15 years from the number on our birth certificate. The more results we see and the younger we feel, the more we enhance the age-nostic lifestyle. It is so much more exciting to feel 40 when you are actually 50!

Some medical practitioners will disagree with the philosophy of age-nostic medicine and some may even describe it as reckless. Indeed, the age-nostic approach does cover a lot of ground that traditional medical practitioners avoid. New medical treatments have always been viewed with suspicion and scepticism, and this is no different. You will also find many medical experts who believe that medical breakthroughs, mainly in the area of hormone replacement therapy and the exciting field of stem cell treatment, will transform the way we age in the coming decades. Real research and studies into anti-ageing treatments are here and further results are coming each year. It is possible to literally reverse the ageing process on a continuous basis. That is what I intend to do and I hope you will as well.

Following the Crowd

Over the years, I have attended many anti-ageing conferences, with some of the larger ones now attended by thousands of doctors. I still seem to be one of the few non-medical people at these events, although I suspect this will change dramatically in the near future. I did have to sign in as a doctor at one show as that seemed the only way to gain access. The lectures and people attending are exactly as a new pioneering belief should be. There is a mix of eccentrics and very non-medical-looking sorts, but the one common feeling is of immense enthusiasm and excitement. I think everyone feels that they are a part of some special club that the majority of people don't know about, and that adds to the electricity.

After I learned as much as I could from others, and in conjunction with some eminent doctors who I shall introduce later, I developed my own protocol and approach. As an example, it took years for me to find a uniform opinion on the amount of human growth hormone I should take. You will hear more about this hormone later in this book. I had settled on the belief that I would get better and safer results by taking less rather than more. I think it was the first major seminar I went to that got me hooked. I have followed the path ever since, and while I used to keep quiet about my exploits and experiments, I now openly talk about age-nostic medicine. This book is partly about my personal journey of discovery and struggle with ageing and life in general as I got older.

It is always wonderful to achieve something after wanting it so badly. However, it is much more satisfying to get something back once you have lost it. Reversing the ageing process through the age-nostic lifestyle is immensely rewarding. Somehow it gives us back what we have lost: the enjoyment and feeling that life is not on the downward spiral but can have upward motion. This sense restores our desire to enjoy life as much as we used to.

We all like to achieve something and live in the best way we can, but as you will see from my personal story, I, like most of us, have suffered from bad decisions both in my lifestyle and in my health. My nature was like many other men: a feeling of invincibility. That gave me license to abuse my body and mind, believing that I could always bounce back. Sadly, the effects of those sorts of choices for most of us don't become apparent until we reach 40 years of age. We wake up one day realizing life and our health are not as they should be and we usually accept the downward spiral as we motor towards 50. I am not a medical doctor or a psychologist – I still probably need one – I am simply a man that wanted to age in a different way and get back the years I felt I had lost through working too hard. I didn't want to find myself hitting the big milestones and experiencing the feeling of a glass half empty, instead of half full.

The Age-nostic Lifestyle

Throughout this book and through many of the contributors, we will talk about an age-nostic lifestyle. Various things go into this, but at its heart is a philosophy and state of mind rather than a list of things to do or take. In a nutshell, it is simply about the struggle that we face with the ageing process as men and what happens when we hit a turning point. The age-nostic approach is about drawing up our own individual battle plan to face our ageing crisis, and how to take back 10 to 15 years in the process.

References to addiction, depression, sex, weight loss, etc. are discussed in depth throughout the whole book because they are key indicators to assess the quality of our life. I believe that for most people to achieve an age-nostic state of mind, they need to consider taking supplements, lose weight, eat the right things, exercise more and become mentally prepared for the problems that arise as we get older, plus look into growth hormones and testosterone replacement to help fight the ageing process. This is not meant to sound too daunting, as you will probably not need all of these things. It is all about finding the right elements that make up your own solution.

Anyone can be age-nostic: they just need to not accept the way we are meant to age and explore the technologies, medicines and help that is now available to us. I am sure in years to come that many of what are called alternative medicines will be commonplace and taken by men as a matter of course. We are the pioneers because we are living in an age where research into the ageing process is in its infancy. Anti-ageing medicine is no longer the playground of the rich, but something that every man can explore without taking out a second mortgage. The right solution to your ageing process isn't on a pharmacy shelf; you have to go and put the bits together. No one knows your body better than you, and the vast majority of the medical profession are concerned about other people rather than your problems. The only driver of this bus is you.

Contributions

You will hear from my good friend, Dr. Michael Zacharia, who 12 years ago asked me to come to a small seminar on anti-ageing medicine. This was an event that would change my life and start me on the journey of testing and questioning the normal way we age. He is a pioneer in this field, and his contribution throughout this book will provide a medical perspective on the treatments and protocols of my own journey into age-nostic medicine, and many other things besides.

You will hear from Tim Watson-Munro, a highly acclaimed psychologist with an international reputation in the field of human behaviour and, in particular, men's self-destruction when the wheels fall off in their lives. I believe that these two professionals will give you a balanced and informed view on the journey I have chosen. You can find out more about Michael and Tim in their biographies in Appendix 1 of this book.

Much of the content in the forthcoming chapters revolves around personal experiences rather than my preachings. I decided to do this for two reasons. First, reading solely about what I might think is right for you is likely to bore even the ardent enthusiast. Second, I am the kind of person who always places more weight on people's real experiences rather than pure theory and hypotheses. The contributors speak from the heart and outline what has happened to them and others around them. In the end, I hope this book will help you to make your personal choice on how you want to go forward. If nothing else, I hope you find it a fascinating journey into what is available if you decide to follow the age-nostic lifestyle.

So Why Change?

So why change the way things are supposed to be? Personally, I have never accepted the way things are meant to be for just about anything. There is something very inspiring about cheating the process. The mere fact that I have experienced such profound results and dared to experiment meant I was challenging the traditional notion of ageing. I was very moved on one occasion when I was discussing the whole subject of anti-ageing with my partner at the time. She believed it was much better to age gracefully. While

I respected her acceptance of the perceived path she was on, I thought it was quite an ironic comment from someone who was still blossoming and glowing with youth. It was a simple assumption but made without fully understanding what was coming in the years ahead. I wonder if she will see it the same way when she approaches her 50th birthday.

Why Just Men?

Discussions have continued about female ageing for many centuries, whereas men have been rather left out in the cold. The female menopause is well documented, but there is very little written or researched about the male mid-life crisis. Men are becoming more aware of their health, performance and appearance than ever before, and the impact of abusing ourselves is more widely understood. I'm not just talking here about drink and drugs, but stress, anxiety, poor diets, depression, addiction and many other things. We have seen a huge increase in cosmetic surgery in women as they attempt to stall the ageing process, but men just seem to get prematurely older. Simply put, most men deserve better access to all the treatments and the critical knowledge on which to base life-changing decisions. That way, more of us can go down the right path or at least understand the options and consequences if we don't.

What Will You Learn From This Book?

Some of the things you will encounter are as follows:

- You will gain an understanding of how hormones have such a dramatic effect on the ageing process and how the decline in levels in our bodies can dramatically affect our mood, sex life and general well-being. You will hear about how topping up these hormone levels will give you back the vitality of your earlier years.
- How depression and other similar mental conditions can be eased and avoided through supplements, lifestyle changes and diet. In many cases, they can be avoided altogether if the signs are picked up early enough. A significant part of the age-nostic approach is helping us become more in tune with what our body and mind are saying. Far too many people start

looking into anti-ageing medicine after a meltdown or major negative event. We want to try to prevent this.

- How to improve your sex life and get back the intimate experiences you thought had abandoned you.
- A new way to lose weight and keep it off, which, in turn, will take years off your appearance, as well as restore confidence and a sense of well-being.
- Supplements that could help to strengthen your mood, vitality and energy.
- How ground-breaking stem cell technology, vitamin drips and injections, which have been enjoyed by Asian men for years, might help you.

The Ageing Process

Much is said and a lot is misunderstood about how we age. We all age differently, but there are some common things that we all experience to a greater or lesser extent. Here is a list of facts.

37 Facts of Ageing

1. Muscle mass decreases and this loss accelerates after age 40.
2. Fat increases as a percentage of body weight.
3. Strength, energy and speed of the body decreases.
4. Basal metabolic rate (metabolism) decreases.
5. Aerobic capacity (the capacity to process oxygen) decreases. Red blood cells, as a percentage of total blood volume (hematocrit) decreases.
6. Body cells become resistant to insulin.
7. LDL cholesterol ("bad" cholesterol) and triglycerides increase, and HDL cholesterol ("good" cholesterol) decreases.
8. Blood pressure increases.
9. Bone mineral density decreases.
10. Kidney functions decrease.
11. We lose neurons in our brain. This can lead to conditions such as Alzheimer's, Parkinson's and senile dementia.
12. Growth hormone secretion decreases.
13. Testosterone levels in men decrease. Oestrogen and progesterone in women decrease.

14. Sexual desire and ability decrease.
15. Thyroid hormone (which affects metabolism) decreases.
16. Melatonin (a hormone that regulates the body clock) decreases.
17. DHEA (a hormone precursor to testosterone and oestrogen) decreases.
18. EPO (erythropoietin, a hormone that stimulates the production of new red blood cells) decreases.
19. Oestradiol, a female hormone, increases in men.
20. Cortisol (often called the "Death Hormone") increases.
21. A bad enzyme, MAO-B, increases in the brain. MAO-B destroys neurons that produce dopamine, which is a neurotransmitter.
22. Aromatase enzyme increases. Aromatase converts testosterone to oestrogen in men, which decreases libido and adds fatty deposits.
23. The thickness of skin decreases, resulting in more wrinkles.
24. Prolactin, a female hormone, increases in the body of a male, depriving him of some of his sexual libido.
25. The water proportion in the body and the skin decreases. This results in (among other things) drier skin and more wrinkles.
26. Sense of hearing decreases.
27. Sense of taste decreases ("Everything tastes the same").
28. Sense of vision, especially capacity to read small letters in low light, decreases.
29. Hair falls and loses its colour (it becomes white).
30. The thymus gland, the master of the immune system, shrinks and atrophies, thus lessening our immune system.
31. Our liver, brain and other critical organs shrink in size, thus affecting their functions.
32. Lipofuscin ("liver spots") accumulates in our hands and our brains. This snuffs out many neurons in the brain.
33. The circulatory system deteriorates in length, width and flexibility, increasing blood pressure and the risk of heart attack.
34. The velocity of blood flow decreases.
35. Inflammation increases in our body.
36. "Deep sleep" becomes scarcer and less profound.
37. Digestion becomes slower and less complete.

I wish you good luck on your journey, especially to those either in the second half of their life or approaching it. Life would be no fun if it was easy, and it certainly doesn't get any easier as we get older. However, I believe there are significant benefits to be had by adopting an age-nostic lifestyle. When I was in my very early 50s, I was evaluated by an anti-ageing doctor who tested how my body was performing. I came out with an age-nostic age of around 35 years. I hope you can do just the same. Most importantly, this book is written by a man who has fallen over more than most, but has managed to keep going and keep faith.

One reason to think about changing now is because anti-ageing itself is coming of age. Up until now, few great medical minds and little money have been put towards research. It has been left in the corner. To put this into perspective, Dr. Michael Zacharia ends this chapter with a personal viewpoint on the early years of anti-ageing treatment and how it has since evolved.

The Early Years of Anti-ageing
By Dr. Michael Zacharia

My experience in anti-ageing medicine started in mid-1997 when I was working in Los Angeles with the famous plastic surgeon, Dr. Harry Glassman. Dr. Glassman had all sorts of interesting patients, but there was one particular patient, Jim, that I remember distinctly. He was in his 60s, had had various surgical procedures, used to arrive at the clinic wearing a singlet and running shorts...he was well known to us all. Jim was the first patient I had met who was taking growth hormone.

At the time, growth hormone was a big mystery and was derived from cow brains. Jim had a document outlining the benefits and explained what it achieved for him personally. This included improved skin tone, lowering body fat and an increased sense of well-being. He was a big fan, and this stimulated me into researching the topic further.

On my return to Australia, I encountered many patients who were keen to improve their inner health as well as their outer appearance. Some patients looked good but felt terrible on the inside, and wanted to make a change for the better. It was in Sydney in September 2001 that I met Dr. Bob Goldman, Chairman of The American Academy of Anti-ageing Medicine. We talked for hours about internal ageing and ways of "stopping the clock", and he invited me to attend the Annual A4M Conference held every December in Las Vegas. Bob had started A4M in 1993 in New York with six doctors including a plastic surgeon, Dr. Vincent Giampapa. Bob had a particular interest in exercise physiology and was the personal fitness adviser to The White House. He still holds many world records relating to fitness. The first A4M Conference in Florida had approximately 15 attendees and two sponsors. By 2001, the meeting shifted to Las Vegas with 4,000 attendees and 300 sponsors. Now it has grown to be even bigger with over 30,000 members worldwide and conferences in more than 15 countries.

In 2002, I began to attend internal medical courses and incorporate anti-ageing medicine into my practice by employing local physicians who were knowledgeable, experienced and passionate in this field. It was in 2002 that I took Michael Hogg along to one of the local anti-ageing conferences and introduced him to the world of longevity medicine.

What is longevity medicine? It is the combination of non-medical and, where necessary, medical therapies to allow us to enter into the second stage of life and live the healthiest and best we can. It is not simply prescribing massive doses of hormones, which has been and still is a common misconception. It is a combination of diet, exercise, relaxation, supplementation, medical treatments and newer genetic treatments to live longer and healthier. It should all start before the age of 40!

There can be no more important start to a long life than diet and exercise. A nourishing diet high in protein but balanced with carbohydrates and fats is vital. Like Bob Goldman, we have been able to look at how to stay fit and healthy through exercise, and this has been a cornerstone in anti-ageing medicine. However, supplementation cannot be underestimated. Where necessary, appropriate medical treatments such as hormone replacement therapies are essential for balancing the internal metabolic orchestra.

As we get older, virtually all of our hormones decrease after peaking in our 20s. Thyroid hormone, oestrogen, testosterone, growth hormone and others all start to reduce as we age. Menopause is well recognized as a result of changes in oestrogen and progesterone levels in women. However, andropause is only just becoming recognized as that change in life in men where the levels of testosterone decrease, with resulting changes in mood, libido and sexual function.

Some of the early treatments in anti-ageing medicine were simply to use hormone therapy. However, as the theories of ageing have developed, so have the intricacies of hormone therapies and the necessity to add lifestyle programmes into any anti-ageing regime. We cannot batter ourselves in the early part of our life with insufficient sleep, poor diet, smoking, recreational drugs, obesity and no exercise, and then expect a miracle Proton Pill to change it all around for us, allowing us to live the second stage healthy and disease-free. We need to start as early as possible, and look after ourselves from a much healthier age, to grow well into the second stage.

Taking supplements has been promoted for years, and I remember reading an article about an 80-year-old man who looked in his 50s and was still fighting fit. He was taking the fat-soluble vitamins A, D, E and K and selenium on a regular basis. There are thousands of articles discussing the pros and cons of vitamin therapy and mineral supplementation, and we know the body yearns for these elements when in poor supply. We also know that giving big doses of intravenous vitamins such as vitamin C has an incredible antioxidant effect, but how significant of an effect can be achieved via the oral route? Supplementation in my mind is essential, and keeping the body topped up regularly is a good start to a healthy lifestyle. When I was 10 years old, I vividly recall asking my great uncle Lauro, who was in his 70s and had fantastic smooth, shiny, full-bodied skin, how he maintained it. He said that since he was 16 he applied moisturizer to his skin immediately after shaving and had done this every day for 60 years. A testament to this is the fact that I have done this myself and continue to have full, healthy skin like my uncle. But uncle Lauro never had access to the new age-nostic therapies.

Nowadays, hormone replacement therapy requires that we look at the symphony of hormones that circulate through our body 24 hours a day. We know a lack or absence of a specific hormone will cause tremendous negative effects on the body; however, what does it mean when that hormone is only lower in the range of normal rather than typical of a disease state? We know thyroid hormone levels have a relationship to vitality, energy, weight and age. Oestrogen and progesterone levels in females change throughout the normal menstrual cycle and then decrease rapidly after menstruation, and their absence can have a huge effect on the female body. Testosterone levels in men fall as we age and may have an effect on energy, mood, libido and sexual function.

The philosophy we follow in our current concept of anti-ageing medicine is to maintain hormone levels in the mid-range for a youthful individual, i.e. if we are 50 years old, we want to maintain our levels similar to that of someone who is 30. Lifestyle, exercise and diet have a significant impact on hormone levels, and we know that regular exercise can lift the natural amount of free testosterone circulating in the body. Another factor we need to consider is that for two individuals of the same age and with the same hormone level, one may not be as responsive to this hormone as the other. Depending on their clinical symptoms, one might require replacement therapy to achieve a certain result, i.e. the testosterone level may be 25 in each 50-year-old man; however, one has poor libido and erectile function whereas the other has the libido and ability of a 30-year-old.

Today, the most significant inroad into anti-ageing medicine is genetic testing and how we deal with telomeres. Genetic testing can be performed using a simple swab taken from the mouth, and then we can look at the DNA makeup of that individual. Specifically, we can look at certain genes and whether they have been turned on or not, and we can make lifestyle changes to affect this switch. We can take a swab of the skin and determine its genetic makeup and the presence or absence of skin-specific genes. With this information we can generate a tailor-made regime to get the skin back to its healthiest, and then monitor progress with further skin gene testing.

Each strand of DNA is paired with another, and they are held together at each end by proteins called telomeres – like the two ends of a shoelace. Every time a cell replicates and divides, so does the DNA; however, after several divisions the telomeres start becoming frayed, like an old shoelace, and this results in the death of that cell. Now we have the capability to monitor the status of our telomeres using a supplement called TA65 to stop them fraying, and possibly extend the life of individual cells. This is probably part of the answer to healthy ageing.

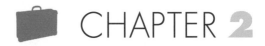

CHAPTER **2**

MY JOURNEY TO AGE-NOSTIC

A rollercoaster career and life

It's 1997, I am 38 and married with two children. One day, I get a call from my close friend, Rob, who tells me his eccentric brother, who is living in Mindanao in the southern Philippines (still a very dangerous place but much more dangerous in 1997), is looking for someone to help him create his business. The region was controlled by Islamic fundamentalists who were effectively the indigenous native population. They had recently gained rights to huge tracts of land that were rich in minerals, especially gold and plantation timber. The gold mining area had long been abandoned by big companies after the fall of the Marcos regime, as well as the constant trouble with militants who had their own formidable army. This meant that no one was interested in commercially mining the area anymore, even though it was, and still is, one of the richest gold belts in the world. I was captivated by the opportunity to go searching for the legendary lost Marcos gold, which was apparently buried in Mindanao by the Japanese at the end of World War II. We eventually went to see this gold after trudging through the jungle with blindfolds accompanied by natives with AK 45s. They had a bizarre plan to ship it to Hong Kong via the sea, but we were the only foreigners down there then and thus their only choice.

I was consulting for a large Malaysian timber company at the time who had bought an Australian firm. I was hired to become the Australian company's marketing director and create a new promotional campaign for the operation. God knows how I got the job, but as usual, it was through my contacts with a couple of very eccentric ex-bankers who did most of their business at lunch. They had an office in one of Sydney's most prestigious buildings, Chifley Tower, which had been built at huge expense by Alan Bond, one of Australia's biggest and most colourful entrepreneurs. This was well before his eventual downfall and prison term. The lunches themselves were great, but I really didn't know anything about timber, and when it was time for me to present my marketing plan to the board of the company, that became very apparent.

So when my friend Rob offered me an opportunity to work on something new in the Philippines, I jumped at the chance. The money was very acceptable and the adventure seemed too good to pass up. I had first met Rob when I was in the hotel and bar business and had hired him as a personal trainer. Rob had graduated from the elite SAS military in Perth, so when he explained the dangers we could face in the Philippines, I was comforted by the fact that he would be by our side. This was to prove very prophetic as the adventure unraveled.

We landed in Manila, a totally chaotic city and far from a "normal" environment. Rob's brother, John, was the closest thing to Indiana Jones I had ever come across; he was a charismatic and charming rogue. Eventually it became impossible to work with John in such a chaotic situation, but Rob and I decided to stay as we had seen and experienced too many amazing things. The chance to do something potentially big and interesting got the better of us. Before we knew it, we had set up our own office deep in Mindanao with some Filipino partners. It always made me nervous that there were hardly any foreigners in this part of the world, and on many occasions we needed heavily armed guards with us.

We focused on obtaining timber poles to electrify the island, and through another contact I obtained 7,000 poles from Canada. We successfully shipped them into the country, which was the first legal foreign shipment to come into Mindanao for many years. This was a grey and murky world. The process to get them in was incredibly complicated, corrupt and risky, as we had to make extra payments to certain people and were never quite sure what would happen from start to end. Creating contracts and paperwork weren't how most people did business, and this often made for a very fluid situation. It certainly kept us constantly in a state of stress.

I was keen not to have all our eggs in one basket. So we spent a lot of time in the jungle deep in militant areas signing up bands of natives to 50/50 joint ventures to develop the old Marcos gold mines. We had huge success establishing a footprint in significant areas, but we couldn't quite work out how to make money. The potential was substantial, but it could all so easily fall completely flat.

Life was taking a very surreal turn, as we were both getting very concerned for our personal safety as well as how the individual deals were going to pan out. We were suddenly hanging out of military helicopters flying over illegal gold mines, wearing military clothes and visiting places we really shouldn't have been going to as foreigners. On one occasion, our geologist from Perth had managed to offend a very influential man at a dinner meeting, and I needed to convince him against shooting his gun in the middle of the restaurant. Our whole lives were taking on an apocalyptic feeling as we lost touch with reality and drifted way out of our depth.

We were dealing with people on a daily basis who would not hesitate to kill us, but we were comforted by the fact that they needed us as no one else was mad enough to be down there. As an example, we received an order for 25,000 telegraph poles, a huge amount in anyone's language, and we knew we would make a substantial amount of money from this order. Through my contacts, I flew to Chile to secure the order. Before I knew it, I was in a private jet heading up the coast from Santiago to meet a timber grower. He lived on a huge estate with a beautiful winery, and suddenly I was touring the vast forest looking at timber, acting as if I knew what I was looking at.

We got on well, and with my sales skills, I convinced him to cut the trees on a very small deposit. We started the process back in Mindanao of getting letters of credit from the electrical company to back the order. We made progress in putting the financial end together and our Chilean partner cut all 25,000 poles, delivering them to the docks in Santiago. And that's when things went very wrong. As foreigners, we couldn't seem to complete the complicated transaction with the various organizations controlling the movement of goods from the port, as there were too many brown paper bags to contemplate; and eventually we were unable to get the poles out of the docks. We lost our $150,000 deposit, and by that time we were completely out of our depth and tired of living on the edge. The Chilean partners were, of course, catatonic with rage as 25,000 poles is a lot of wood, and our Filipino partners were not happy at the state of the transaction.

After multiple threats and one man turning up to my apartment with a very large gun, I decided to make a graceful, if speedy, exit from the country. I said I was going to the shops but went straight to the airport and have never been back since. I had moved my family to Bali as it was too dangerous to live in the Philippines, and I suddenly found myself back in Sydney facing some angry investors with no more than a hundred dollars to my name. The experience was beginning to take its toll. I was not in good mental shape at all, and I knew I had to get back on my feet quickly. I took the first job I could, as an assistant manager in a well-known restaurant in Sydney based on my experience gained in my own hospitality businesses. The pay was minuscule, but it was working and I quickly took to it. After a few months, I got my family back to Australia and was able to look forward again.

I could never say I am an orthodox guy with an orthodox career and life. My adventures in the Philippines are clear proof of that. In fact, my whole life journey to where I am now has been a rollercoaster ride, as I have tried desperately to keep the ball rolling. My story is probably an extreme one by most standards, but I believe no one's life and career is smooth and predictable. I want to tell you my journey because it is proof that if someone as erratic and unorthodox as me can do it, then so can most men.

My childhood was relatively normal most of the time. I was always the one who talked too much in class and was never interested in studies except art, which may have been fuelled by having a crush on the female art teacher. Art was the only subject I channeled any effort into, and after 10 years of expensive school fees, I failed totally. The only transferable skill seemed to be the ability to be enthusiastic about almost anything. My school report marks were so bad that I used to wait at the mailbox and steal them before my parents had time to read them.

My school was the first boys' school in Sydney that would accept girls, but even then only in my last two years. I remember the day all these beautiful creatures came through the front gates, which didn't help our marks at all. In the last year of school, my history teacher approached me to say his brother had an advertising agency and was looking for a graduate with some special skills. As it was the time of the "mad men" era, I definitely thought that advertising, or business on the whole, was just going to lunch, smoking and drinking a great deal. So I was the perfect candidate, with all the right credentials.

I was just about to start the job in January 1978 and had gone skiing before tackling the unsuspecting corporate world head-on. After a night partying, I smashed my leg and fractured it right up to my knee. The first day of my new job, my mother had to drive me to the office and I walked through reception on crutches. Like most things in my early life, the job didn't last long.

I was 18 and not really interested in work or many aspects of grown-up life. So I did the usual thing and headed off to Europe, with a one-way ticket ending up in London's Earls Court, because that's where all the Australians seemed to be hanging out. I had the normal adventures heading to Greece and remember getting off at Corfu on the way to Athens for just one day. I met a girl that night and didn't get back on board for another three months. We had a wonderful time together in spite of different language skills, but eventually she had to leave the island. We agreed to meet in Paris on a particular day in about four weeks, but in the end, I was having too much fun and didn't turn up. I felt guilty for decades about how I let her down.

Eventually, I returned from Europe with no money in my pocket and quickly got a job as a night porter in a three-star hotel. Luckily I learned quickly that if you are prepared to work hard, you can make money. My love of nomadic adventure got me interested in the travel industry, and I quickly talked my way into a number of jobs without any real experience. I always got bored and my lack of attention to detail didn't prove to be a great quality. One job proved to be the last straw, when I forgot to book a family onto a cruise trip. By the time my boss had found the unbanked cheque in my drawer, it was too late to book the family on the trip as the cruise of a lifetime was full. Again, this was a hard lesson to learn as I had really let people down, myself included.

I was not built to be a travel agent. I just didn't have the patience or attention span to be successful at that time, and my only claim to fame was having a brief affair with the prettiest girl in the agency. This caused all sorts of trouble for me, but that didn't stop me from focusing on what I wanted. Because I was confident and knew how to talk, I then secured one of the best jobs around, as a sales representative at a major airline. The job was to visit travel agents and promote the airline that was constantly full. In those days, 90% of travel agents were made up of young females, and I could fill a book with the adventures I enjoyed. In any case, after a while, I realized this job was going nowhere.

Nothing Ever Goes to Plan

Being in the right place at the right time should never be underestimated. A friend was sailing a 70-foot long ketch to Perth for the 1987 Americas Cup. He was looking for crew so, aged 26, I jumped at the chance to have some fun, get away from everything and make a new start. I arrived in Perth and spent the entire Americas Cup period sailing, having fun and working on the boat with not a care in the world. Fremantle, which is very close to Perth, was where the Cup was being held, and it was the most exciting place in the world at that time. We were fit and tanned and life was sailing by day and partying by night. Things were really looking up.

And then it was suddenly over in a flash as Australia lost the Cup, and Fremantle changed from a place of international excitement to a sleepy ghost town. Like a lot of people in their 20s today, planning ahead wasn't really on my radar. I decided to go back to Sydney as I was feeling homesick for the first time in my life. I needed to get some money together first, and managed to get a job working as the sales manager in a big hotel. There wasn't much excitement or stimulation, so I was getting progressively more bored as the days went on. One of my work colleagues had invited me to a charity dinner on a Saturday night, but at 6pm I was happy to sit on the couch after a busy week, assessing what the next move should be. My colleague came to my apartment and forced me to get dressed. I walked into the function and there were eight people at one particular table. I immediately noticed a striking-looking girl at the end.

Somehow I made up the ninth person and ended up next to her. I was talking away and she was looking at me with a bemused look on her face. She did her best to ignore me but I couldn't forget meeting her and became very focused. The next day, I sent her some flowers with the message, "Lovely to meet you last night". I got up the courage to ask her out, which she reluctantly agreed to. She had the same look on her face all night and I couldn't work it out. She was obviously intrigued but wasn't sure what kind of guy I really was. However, after much debate and plenty of persuasion, we married nine months later. We had 18 years of marriage together and have two beautiful children.

From Philippines to Sydney

After leaving the madness of the Philippines, I started to put out feelers to get back to Sydney. That was where I could make things happen, achieve some meaningful momentum and get some deals going. My brother helped me start a small call centre that turned quickly into a more significant business, which in 1999 was just before the Internet boom. The economy was growing and I felt many businesses needed a better customer service proposition. We purchased a piece of software that was a forerunner to automated email, which of course now is part of everyday life. When I look back, it is amazing what can be done when you put your mind to it and want something badly enough. I needed to get my family back together and establish a solid home for them, especially after my Philippines debacle. All of this happened in the space of 12 months, and I went from having almost nothing in the bank to running my own successful business.

Our big break came when the software we bought created some interest from a couple of big players. An old friend of mine, who ran one of the biggest insurance companies down under, agreed to invest in the company. He and one of Australia's most successful business families agreed in principle to invest $2,000,000 into our company, and we had a great article in the *Australian Financial Review* as a result. Having the business family on our side was going to be a huge help, as they owned controlling interests in TV and newspapers. They were also involved in gambling, tourism and other industries besides. It was these connections that made the deal exciting for me as it opened doors that would otherwise have been firmly shut.

However, Lady Luck was about to turn her back on me. The 2000 tech crash hit us hard. The business family pulled their investment out and we couldn't afford to keep the infrastructure we had created going for long without a sizeable cash injection. A few months later, we had to wind the company up. An earlier article on our company in the Australian press was to change my life and put me on a path that leads to writing this book today. From that article and through another coincidence, I was contacted by an amazing businessman, Chris, who is still today the closest thing to a mentor I have ever had. Chris had started out in the late 80s creating a direct sales business with a couple of friends in a small apartment in Sydney. He primarily started selling books door-to-door. Today, the company operates in 22 countries and has over 10,000 full-time sales staff.

We met for lunch, something he rarely does, and his incredible enthusiasm and drive totally captivated me. Besides him being one of the most caring and honest people I have ever met, he has also given thousands of young people a chance to learn skills and build the first step towards a career. He is an amazing man who optimized the belief that you can start with nothing and build a huge company. More importantly, his philosophy was to share the rewards with everyone who works hard and sticks at it. I learned a great deal from this guy. The door-to-door industry is often perceived badly, but it gave many young people skills and a job where their own efforts were rewarded. Chris is an amazing salesperson and has one of the best intellects I know. He is not interested in the day-to-day running of the business and still spends much of his time with the sales teams. Being at the sharp end is where he still wants to be.

I helped him restructure the company and loved the excitement that sales brought. The young people we worked with were mostly in their 20s, bringing their enthusiasm and youthful energy to make anything possible. I had found my niche at the age of 41 years. I had been given a real chance and working with Chris was a good fit for me. I threw myself into the job because the enthusiasm around me was amazing. I have never turned around a company of this size but I had my family settled and my kids back at a good school. I felt fortunate to have been given this chance (especially considering my track record), so I worked hard and took advantage of my luck.

I did a good job because I really wanted the company and the people to succeed. I was getting results, and it wasn't long before Chris asked me to go to Europe because his business had expanded so much that he was having trouble managing the growth. In reality, this meant keeping the costs in check while trying to expand the company base. The funny thing is, I had no financial experience or training and am not great with my own finances. But never one to take a backward step, I relished the role and learned very quickly how to make a difference. Through making some very tough decisions, we turned the company around in a relatively short period. We flattened the management hierarchy and focused everyone on what our customers wanted. The results were immediate and soon made the company healthy and more profitable.

One of the best days of my business life was when Chris got up at a sales rally in front of over 3,000 people and said that without me, we would all not be here today. I felt like I was at the height of my career.

Life is Not Just About Business

I don't really like this heading, because for me it sums up many of my mistakes as I was going through my 30s and 40s. But I decided to keep it to remind me what life is really not all about: it is not all about business. Yet, for most of my adult life, I was convinced it was.

Like many men from my era, life was all about a career. Or perhaps it was really all about approval and, dare I say, ego. In my case, I did badly at school and never went to university, so it was simply a case of proving to others (although not to myself) that I was capable of achieving something. I think for men in general, the approval and endorsement of others drives many of us in directions we would never dream of going (or indeed should ever go, because it simply does not match up to who we are or who we should become). For many men, this can have devastating effects as we reach maturity in our business life and career. We end up hitting the panic button because of what I call the "too late syndrome".

During the writing of this book, I bumped into my hairdresser on the tube. It was uncanny because I was just about to ring her to book in a trim. I had just come out of a particularly bad bout of depression after some terrible news and far too much travel. This combination caused the usual self-medication and guilt I feel when coming off my path of age-nostic living. I had not exercised for a few days, had eaten badly and had not slept well. Fortunately, it was reasonably short-lived and I was soon getting back to where I should be.

As my hairdresser and I sat in the tightly cramped tube train, we started talking about how my writing was going (I had mentioned the book project briefly to her during one of our sessions). She wanted to know more about the book. I explained it was about being a man and growing older and how to accept certain downsides, but not to accept the traditional ageing process. I went on to talk about the three big subjects of addiction, depression and relationship breakdown. Whenever I do that, it always seems to start most women talking as if I am the partner they lost or was with or they wanted to meet, and this conversation on the tube was no different.

She told me there was a study about boys and girls of a very young age and how significantly the boys reacted to a situation of confrontation or perceived danger. The study revealed that the girls did little but stare, and the boys in most cases wanted to run away in fear. In a few cases – called the "warrior response" – some boys faced the situation head-on. There is no doubt that fear drives men much more than security. Men's fear of failure in particular can cause enormous problems. Instead of facing it, too many men run away and look for something else that they can succeed in. For the lucky ones, this can be a new job or career, but often the end result is addiction, relationship breakdown, financial problems or even total meltdown and depression.

As males, our biggest mentor figure tends to be our father. From an early age, most of us worship him and look to him for direction on many important aspects of our life. He is a beacon as we grow through our early years and move into adulthood. He represents a path that many of us decide to follow. We have followed, often subconsciously, many of his career decisions, been attracted to women similar to what he has chosen, and have had comparable ideals. In many cases, way before we have even realized the mistakes he may have made, we are already down a well-worn path.

When we reach our 40s, many of our critical life decisions have been made and we often feel that our life is set on a path we cannot change. We are often reminded of the possible mistakes we have made following our first mentor as we struggle with our own marriages, families, social lives and careers. It is at this time that we are much more likely to go through some sort of panic, thinking our choices were maybe not ours at all.

Some of our health issues later in life can be traced back to parental attitudes or behaviour: if they drank too much, we will tend to do the same; if they ate badly, we will tend to do the same; if they were depressed, we will tend to get depressed. As you will see later in this book, I have periodically suffered from depression and alcohol abuse, something that ran in the family. In a later chapter, Tim Watson-Munro will outline the deep psychological effect our fathers have on our later life as we reach middle age and go through what some call a "mid-life crisis".

There are medical experts who believe many of our negative traits are somehow genetically or chemically set in motion before we are born. I am personally convinced that many of the things we experience early in our life help shape our behaviour later. This only intensifies as we reach the age when our fathers showed their own symptoms.

Before we all become horrified as we review our own life and the bad habits that we have contracted from our major mentor, we should remember that many of our best traits are also installed in us at an early age. Much of our success, solid values and human qualities come from our father. Of course, the influence of our mothers and the kind of interaction our parents had with each other also play an important role. Both of our parents have tremendous influence on the level of happiness, or lack thereof, we experience in our own close partnerships.

The good news is that unless your mother was a clone of Bette Davis and your father was like Ernest Hemingway or Adolf Hitler, most of us will lead relatively happy lives. The important point to note is that if one can simply identify with the theory that many of our beliefs, thoughts and patterns are not really our own, we can then change many of the bad traits that seem to intensify as we grow through our 40s and 50s. The age-nostic lifestyle requires a radical change in our mindset and behaviour. It's not an easy quick-fix. But if you are reading this book and are in your 30s, 40s or 50s, you are in a unique position to change most aspects of the ageing process for the better.

Our own fathers never had access to the technology, knowledge and medical research that we have today and will have in the future. I find it hard to imagine my own father injecting growth hormones, having a regular testosterone shot, taking supplements and keeping his fridge full of concoctions that make it look like a laboratory experiment. That sight has been left for my own children to experience now with fascination and pride as they constantly compare me to their friends' 50+ year-old fathers. Even though I have children who are all grown up now, I marvel at what might be possible through medical progress in the next 10 to 20 years. This will undoubtedly make their ageing process a whole different experience than what they could have expected.

Always Moving Forward

Many people from tough beginnings or the wrong side of the tracks have gone on to do great things. The experiences I had from an early age certainly challenged me to grow up very fast and not to fear what comes straight at us. For me, some of my early life taught me that I needed to use every skill I had to get ahead, and being able to communicate well with people from all walks of life was a great asset. I'm not sure I was naturally born top of the class in anything, but being able to talk with people face-to-face proved helpful again and again.

Ultimately, I have always put great faith in the ability to just keep going, no matter what obstacles are in the way. It is so easy as we get older to find reasons to hit the pause button, to halt the forward momentum, whether in our personal or business lives.

My own business hero was Aristotle Onassis, and I still think that his is one of the best business stories ever told. I am ashamed to say that I paid $5,000 for a letter written by Onassis together with his business card, which are at least extremely rare. After the war, when Onassis had no money at all, he realized that there were hundreds of ships lying around not being used and liked the idea of starting a shipping company (he was Greek, after all). He wanted to ship tobacco from Brazil, as smoking had just become very fashionable and he saw a huge market. He didn't have any money and the bank wouldn't lend him any. He was rejected on numerous occasions regardless of the great tan, great jacket and very small office with a great address. So what he did was sign a series of huge contracts with tobacco suppliers even though he didn't have any way of shipping the goods because he had no ships! He then went to the bank with the contracts and got the money he needed. Cash in hand, he bought the ships. On the basis of this deal he would create the world's largest shipping company from scratch. He would also become the world's richest man.

Many of us read numerous books on goal setting and business planning, but in reality few of us do as much as we should. I am also an avid reader of motivational books and enjoy them with great enthusiasm. They have helped open the door to a new world for me, which is one more organized and focused. But I'm not quite sure why we end up buying so many books every year which basically tell us what we already know deep down. We want to be happy every minute of the day, we want to have eternal good health, we want to be rich, and we want to meet and fall in love with an understanding and beautiful person. Not much to ask for!

One night I was up watching TV and I purchased Anthony Robbins' "Unleash the Power Within" CD series. It was very late at night and it seemed the answer to my state of mind. I called the number and was willing to pay anything to find some happiness. I had forgotten completely about that evening, because some weeks later a CD collection turned up at my office and I could not quite remember ordering it. However, I am an admirer of Anthony Robbins, even though I have never followed the instructions to eternal happiness and riches. I didn't put anything into action straight away, but as with many of these products, it somehow energized me to move forward in a positive way at a time when everything was burning down and falling apart. It gave me something positive to think about and that helped right away. Thank you, Anthony.

About this time I met two brilliant entrepreneurs who were to teach me so much by changing my outlook on work and showing me how to start a company from a garage. Their business was called Matilda Bay Brewery and it brewed beer not far from the centre of Perth. They were becoming highly successful, having built a major boutique brewery and a series of great hotels that broke the mold. They sold their own beers and introduced good food in places with attractive décor. They were pioneers and were to later sell their business to Bond Brewing, which was originally started by Alan Bond and a brand which is still very significant today.

One of the founders noticed my work as a barman and saw some potential. He asked why I was just working behind the bar, having got hold of my résumé. He asked me if I wanted to be assistant manager at one of his hotels after I convinced him that being a sales manager was similar. There may have been a little exaggeration there. I worked hard in record time and loved running a hotel. All the people you meet and learning how to organize many different tasks at once gave me a great insight into what running a business was really like. I loved it and my career was about to go places, which was about time as I was well into my 30s and beginning to feel like an under-achiever.

Another huge influence was my uncle. I became a fitness fanatic because around the age of 12, I had the coolest uncle imaginable. He was a saxophone player, champion boxer and kept himself superbly fit by going to the gym. He loved boxing, and this was in the early 70s when gyms were not what they are today. I never recall seeing my own father do any real exercise at all. His passion was golf, which I am sure was actually a reason to escape my mother and the responsibilities of work. Bringing up a family and many of life's challenges for a man in his late 30s and early 40s in the 60s and 70s was not easy for him.

I remember my cool uncle putting boxing gloves on me and my brother, and while I had a happy relationship with my brother, there was obvious rivalry. Although I don't recall the result of the bout, I do remember the fierceness and passion when we boxed. My uncle also took me out for my first drink (not a good thing, looking back). To me, he was a real life hero and mentor all rolled into one. He gave me the belief that life was an adventure to have and that we never had to act our age just because we were supposed to. Some 40 years later, I believe that he set in motion at the age of 12 the desire in me to stay young and not follow my own relatives into early and premature old age.

Reaching the Land of Age-nostic

It was in 2002 when I went to my first talk on anti-ageing medicine. It was held in Sydney and only around 20 people attended. I had been researching the subject for a while so I had enough basic knowledge to realize that I simply wanted to know more. It was at this talk that I first heard about human growth hormone (HGH) and testosterone treatment for men, and how it could rejuvenate and roll back the clock. As I had just passed the magic milestone of 40, had been married for 10 years, had two young children and very little financial security, I was more than eager to look into the whole anti-ageing philosophy to help secure a better future.

One of the factors that helped spur me down the anti-ageing path was the feeling that at the age of 40, I was behind others. Peers had greater material possessions, career stability and other things. I had always kept myself fit, but wanted to feel 40 when I reached 50.

By 2008, I had been global CEO for a big international company for almost eight years. I was living between London and Sydney, one month each for almost four years, and was regularly visiting another 10 to 15 countries at the same time. I was the last to see it, but the pressure, hours and travel were taking their toll. I was successful in many ways, and had achieved my ambition some years before by coming back from a seemingly impossible position. I had a beautiful home in Sydney, a farm and investment properties, but despite all this success and wealth, I was in trouble and knew it. I was having a mid-life crisis, although I wasn't quite sure what that was.

My marriage collapsed completely, which was totally my fault. I left home one day, rang Chris and told him I couldn't do it anymore. He, of course, was totally compassionate and understood I had burnt out. He knew long before that day, but stuck with me. I had become interested in anti-ageing medicine some years before, and experimented with many different things to slow down the ageing process. Much of what follows in this book is about what I have learned and experienced along this journey. I certainly believe I could not have achieved what I have without being in good shape, both inside and out. But I am far from perfect, and I went through my own periods of being very much the opposite.

Ten Tips for Your Age-nostic Journey

Each chapter in this book will end with a series of 10 tips to help you come to terms with the subject of the chapter. Even if you only follow these tips and nothing else, you will be well on your way to becoming an age-nostic man. Here are the first ones:

1. It's never too late to change.
2. Don't get trapped in something you are not happy doing.
3. Don't stay when you know it's time to go.
4. Don't let your age stop you from chasing your dreams.
5. Never let those around you say you are too old to take risks.
6. Kids are important, but so are you.
7. Don't let money rule your life and stop you taking risks.
8. Don't let your father's fears become your own.
9. If you hate what you are doing, put a plan together to do something new.
10. You still have a choice.

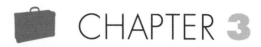

CHAPTER **3**

THE HUMAN GUINEA PIG

How anti-ageing treatments have changed my life

Each human body is different and there is no singular set regime that will work for everyone. I would not expect my regime to work for all males over 40 years of age, but much of it can help the vast majority. I do feel, as do many of my doctor friends and specialists in anti-ageing, that how my body has reacted to certain drugs and treatments is not unusual. This chapter will therefore set out what I have tried and how I have responded physically and mentally. Before going too far with this potentially life-changing journey, I would recommend everyone to have all the tests possible in an attempt to really understand where they are in the ageing process.

The world of anti-ageing medicine is still relatively new, and one of my early frustrations was the conflicting advice I received from both medical practitioners and the written material on the subject. I had met with many of the leading doctors at various conferences around the world and wanted to find out as much as I could about what to take, what was new and what results they were getting with their patients. Because of the relative age of this medical discipline, there was often little real consensus, but trends on results were becoming stronger as we all learned what combinations of things worked best for what kind of individual.

At the end of the lectures at that first anti-ageing conference I attended, I put my hand up to ask the only question I wanted to ask. As is typical in these things, people are more interested in getting to the tea and coffee than delving a little deeper. A doctor on the panel noticed my hand up and I proceeded to stand and say, "Sounds great, where do I get some?" Everyone seemed to turn around and look at me at once as if I had openly asked for a suitcase full of marijuana or cocaine. I didn't really get an answer, except that many of the drugs were a little difficult and complicated to obtain, though not illegal. There was a lot of mystery and reluctance among the medical fraternity, and very few doctors had both the knowledge and willingness to administer these new wonder treatments. That made me even more determined to find out how I could get hold of these "youth elixirs", and it was not going to take me long to get what I wanted. In fact, it took about 10 minutes.

I approached the doctor giving one of the lectures and arranged to visit her surgery the following week. Before this, I had experimented with natural growth hormone releasers, which really had very little impact on me. I worked out that you could take certain amino acids, which come in powder form and are available from most good health food stores. If you take them before going to bed, growth hormone is released at its highest level while we sleep.

I obtained the three amino acids, which had to be mixed with water, although the taste and smell were still simply horrible. It reminded me of those Chinese herbs you mix up when you want a natural cure for a cold. Mind you, they had saved me from an emergency appendix operation in Singapore a few years ago. I had what was later confirmed as appendicitis, but found out I had let my medical insurance lapse and it was incredibly expensive to have the operation in Singapore. I went to the doctor and he said I should go to the hospital. I lived near Chinatown and so headed down to the nearest Chinese doctor. She seemed to know everything about appendicitis, showing me diagrams in a Chinese medical book.

I was in a lot of pain and she spoke no English at all. An extremely attractive receptionist was there to help who had studied in Australia and who spoke perfect English. She translated everything, and while trying to flirt, I understood that I had to take some herbs and cook up some things that looked like a bunch of tree twigs. Two days later, I was completely without pain, and while my appendix was to finally burst in London some 18 months later, I was glad that the treatment worked and I didn't have to pay for an expensive operation in Singapore. (In London, after I did eventually have my appendix out, I was supposed to remain in hospital for longer, but decided to check myself out early. During the next week, I took sheep placenta injections and increased my growth hormone intake. Now, since I am not a qualified doctor, this is my own opinion: my recovery was incredible and very quick. Even my friends could not quite believe it. But I could clearly see my recovery was aided by my age-nostic lifestyle.)

Back to my journey. I tried mixing the concoction for about a week, late at night, making a huge mess in the kitchen with all this white powder all over the place. I remember my wife coming downstairs looking at me and, as usual, never making a comment or complaining. She had already become used to some of my eccentric ways and new ideas, and I am sure she was thinking this was just another manic obsession that would soon pass.

I quickly decided that I neither had the discipline nor the patience to continue on the path of creating my own mixtures, and I was making a hell of a mess in the kitchen each night. I realized that I had to find another way, and had recently finished reading a fantastic book called *Grow Young with HGH* by Ronald Klatz. I had read it all in one night and then trawled the net to find if there was an alternative. Finally, I found a site in America that looked reputable (not a hard thing to do on the net). They sold a fizzy tablet called "Pro-HGH", which expounded that it could mimic the results of taking injectable HGH. I ordered some straight away. I had expected customs to turn up with it at the door, as Australia has very strict import laws, but they probably didn't understand what it was.

I started taking the tablets as advised. They were really just like taking a Berocca, and the manufacturers were smart enough to make them taste great as well. Who really knew whether the stuff worked, but I was on my journey and excited, and wanted more. I followed this regime religiously for about a month, but as I continued to research the subject, I came to the conclusion that if I really wanted to obtain the best results, I had to go "full monty". That was to obtain a pharmaceutical injectable synthetic HGH. There is no one more fearful of injections than myself, mainly due to those giant injections dentists had in the late 60s. I went to the doctor I had seen before, and had blood tests done to check my levels of growth hormones. I received my test results, and while my levels were not critically low, I decided by choice to start the injections to see if it was possible to reverse them back to a level at least 10 years younger than my biological age.

I was reading many articles that did not agree with taking HGH, saying that it caused all types of side effects and may even cause cancer. However, I had met many leading world experts who had written numerous articles saying the exact opposite. To me, it was a personal choice and the positive effects of increasing levels of HGH far outweighed any negative research. I also felt that when anything new came around in medicine, there was always a proportion of insiders who were afraid of change and would blindly back the status quo. I certainly felt that taking the right level of compounds was crucial, but that is something that is different for each person.

As a slight aside, I remember some years ago a famous American actor was detained at Sydney Airport for bringing in vials of HGH. As he was only in Sydney for a short period, I was amazed at the amount he had with him and I was only taking a fraction of what he must have been consuming. Like any other pharmaceutical drug, it will cause side effects and is potentially damaging if you take it in the wrong dose. Taking relatively small amounts to top up your own levels seemed to be the right approach.

My regime was to take a small amount for five days using a very small injection similar to a diabetic needle, then take two days off. I have been doing that for 12 years now and have achieved the results that the research promised. When I was young, I used to get quite a few colds and have only had two in the last 12 years: those only lasted a day at most. My health in my 40s and early 50s is vastly better than in my 20s and 30s. I have fewer mood swings, better energy levels, better skin tone and generally better everything. It took about six months to really feel the effects, but they were profound. Over the years, I have taken breaks, usually about four to six months, but the difference has been so obvious that I have always been eager to get back onto my regime.

Besides HGH, my treatment and supplement regime today consists of the following:

- Peptides
- KH3 and GH3
- Placenta
- B12 shots
- IV drip
- Stem cells
- 5HTP
- Aminoguanidine
- Carnosine
- CoQ10
- Deprenyl
- DHEA
- Growth hormone
- Hydergine
- Melatonin
- Modafinil
- Oxytocin
- Piracetam
- Testosterone
- Vitamin C
- Vitamin D
- Zinc

Arresting and reversing the ageing process has been my goal when experimenting and finding out the key age-nostic solutions to help me live a better life as I age. You can find numerous articles and comments by experts who do not recommend any of these treatments, and some will say they are dangerous. The lack of long-term studies is the biggest barrier to full endorsement. However, those are difficult to produce since this is a new science and many aspects haven't been around for long. I have made the personal choice to start now and not wait for the research endorsement to be produced, as I will simply be too old for it to make that much difference.

What I can say is the anti-ageing community is much bigger than you could imagine, and I am far from unique in undertaking these treatments. I have no doubt a huge proportion of the people working in Hollywood, on Wall Street and the top end of business executives are also helping themselves with some of these treatments and drugs. The reason we don't hear much about it is that currently it is just not acceptable to tell the world about it.

My view on all of this is very simple. I don't want to age like the generation before me. I want to live with plenty of energy, enthusiasm and excitement way after 50 years of age, and quite frankly I don't see enough men enjoying that opportunity. I hope the description of my regime and the results I am getting will at least make you think of how you want to age. No matter how much money or success you have achieved, or maybe still want to achieve, there is no point whatsoever to it if you are feeling old, depressed and no longer enjoying life to the full.

New age-nostic treatments are becoming available as you read this book. One of those is peptides, which I recently discovered and have started using to good effect. Dr. Michael Zacharia provides here an overview of this amino acid and how it works.

An Overview on Peptides
By Dr. Michael Zacharia

Our bodies are made up of various forms of amino acids. In fact, our genetic makeup of DNA is a double-chain spiral of amino acids. A peptide is a short chain of amino acids usually less than 50 in number. When the number is greater than 50, the compound becomes a protein or a polypeptide. The interesting thing about peptides is that because they are so small, they can be delivered into the human body in oral, cream or injectable forms. This is unlike human growth hormone, which is a polypeptide comprising a chain of 191 amino acids and is so large it can only enter the body by injection.

Peptides can stimulate or mimic what other normal active proteins in the body do. For example, Melanotan 2 is a peptide, which stimulates the melanocytes in the skin to produce and release more melanin. As a result, the skin becomes tanned and might even provide a protective barrier to UV light. As an aside, Melanotan 2 also has an aphrodisiac effect and can stimulate spontaneous erections.

In the world of anti-ageing medicine, peptides are gaining a significant profile. For example, CJC-1295 is a peptide (aka growth hormone releasing hormone), which binds to receptors in the pituitary gland and stimulates the release of endogenous growth hormone. It also has anti-inflammatory effects and can promote sleep. Similarly, GHRP6 (growth hormone releasing peptide) stimulates the release of growth hormone from the pituitary but also has an effect on increasing appetite.

AOD9604 HGH Frag 176-191 is a peptide, which simulates the fat-reducing effects of HGH, but only comprises the last 10% of the 191 amino acid chain. As a result, it stimulates lipolysis (the breakdown of fat) and prevents lipogenesis (the formation of fat) without the negative effects on insulin resistance or blood sugar levels. This is a simple small-chain peptide that can be delivered as a cream or injection and has an incredible effect on fat metabolism and body shape and size. There are many other peptides which have beneficial effects on several biological systems in the body, and new peptides are being discovered daily.

I am getting similar results with peptides to those described by Dr. Michael Zacharia but more pronounced, especially with muscle tone and lean body mass. I should point out that while I have been taught to eat well and have always exercised, mainly through vanity, I had also lived under enormous stress, drank far too much at times and still struggled with smoking from time to time. I travelled long distances constantly and generally pushed myself to the limit.

During the 12-year period leading up to writing this book, I have been regularly taking many other supplements and treatments. With everything that I take religiously, I am always very aware of potential side effects. However, I can honestly say that during this journey, the only side effects I have experienced are great health, high levels of energy and confidence.

KH3 and GH3

KH3 (sometimes called GH3) was among the first anti-ageing treatments available and was perfected by a Romanian doctor, Ana Aslan, in the 1960s. It was very popular with the Hollywood set at that time, with the likes of Marlene Dietrich, Salvador Dali and President J. F. Kennedy reported to have taken it. I take KH3 every day in tablet form, which you can get under prescription in most countries. It is not an anti-depressant but definitely has an effect on my mood by providing a general feeling of well-being. In Germany, KH3 is the most popular anti-ageing supplement used.

Sheep placenta

I had heard about this treatment which is usually taken by injection, but being a Kiwi by birth, I was already hearing the jokes from my family and friends. I was amazed at the size of the industry, especially in Asia, mainly among the wealthy Chinese. Most of the high-quality product is made in Switzerland by a few very large companies. It is simply administered over about a month and appears it could help with rejuvenation.

After researching this treatment and its claimed benefits, I was excited to try it. The issue was where to find a reliable supply. When I was in Bali and looking at setting up an age-nostic clinic, I met a doctor who was administering injections. I had also discovered a company in Singapore who had a very high-profile clinic in the most prestigious hotel. The trouble was they were charging $15,000 for one 10-day treatment. Eventually I was to obtain the same treatment from Switzerland through my usual network of doctors.

It needs to be injected into a main muscle group by a doctor. I obtained enough for a three-month course and got a network of doctors (because I was travelling a lot as usual) to administer the correct dose over the period. I felt the effects after the first week: increased energy levels without feeling hyperactive. Also, I quickly felt an increased sense of general well-being and I definitely noticed an improvement in my skin. My only frustration now is the difficulty of transporting it into many countries and that it is quite expensive. For most men, injecting sheep placenta is probably not the first thing to try: it is well down the age-nostic lifestyle road.

Placenta
by Dr. Michael Zacharia

Placenta treatments have been used for many years and are thought to increase energy, vitality, treat liver disease, improve the youthful appearance and possibly help with anti-ageing. They can be sourced from sheep, cows and humans and may be presented as creams, tablets and injections. The active components of placenta are cytokines, enzymes, growth factors, hormones, nutrients and immune system components. We don't know exactly how placenta treatments work, but ask anyone that has used them and they say the result makes them feel generally good. Immediately after their infusion or injection, patients seem to feel better and some of the less prominent problems of ageing, including skin quality, general health and fatigue, seem to improve.

B12 shots
These shots have been around seemingly forever and are now becoming popular among entertainers and corporate high-fliers. There has been some negative press recently caused by some celebrity entertainers, although I doubt whether B12 has been the primary cause of their problems. I get an injection once a month, mainly to help with the number of different time

zones I find myself in. Lots of airline travel doesn't always mean I eat the right balance of food, which can be quite destabilizing in itself. There is no doubt that this simple injection taken in a muscle can be quite painful, but only for a second or two. I feel it is well worth it, especially if you are not getting the right amount of vitamin B. I find it is a great help when fighting against tiredness and low energy or when you are feeling just plain run-down.

IV drip

I also have an IV drip once per month, which is essentially a large dose of vitamin C together with antioxidants. It is inserted into the main vein in my arm and takes about 40 minutes to run through. It is great for getting vitamin C into the system where tablets really don't have the effect they should. I take it during winter to protect against colds, flu and viruses.

Stem cells

I have injected stem cells through an IV drip under medical supervision. Also, because I am losing my hair, they were injected into my scalp. Here's a more detailed explanation of this treatment.

Stem Cells

By Dr. Michael Zacharia

Stem cell treatments are gaining greater popularity for the use of improving general health, for rejuvenation, and more recently to treat disease processes. A stem cell is an originator cell of the body, an undifferentiated cell found among differentiated cell tissue such as fat. These cells are special because they can divide into other types of cells and help to maintain and repair tissue.

There was controversy in the early years of stem cell research and treatments because we only had embryonic stem cells available (i.e. those derived from an embryo). Their use brought about significant religious and ethical issues, and thus stem cell treatments were hard to originate. The only centres available were in China, the Bahamas and Russia. However, those receiving the embryonic cells remarked that their general health, lack of illness and youthfulness were remarkable. These treatments were given intravenously three to four times per year, but were outrageously expensive.

Nowadays, it is a very different matter. We can harvest adult stem cells from our own bodies with the knowledge that these will differentiate into other cells and possibly provide repair of body tissue. Stem cells exist in the blood in low levels and in the bone marrow in high levels. A liposuction procedure can be performed, gathering 100ml of fat and treating it with enzymes to remove all the tissue except for the stem cells. These stem cells are not modified in any way and so governments are not concerned about their use. Several Western governments deem it illegal to manipulate (expand) stem cells once they are outside of the body. This can all be performed in a matter of a few hours in an accredited facility.

Once we have the stem cells, what can we do with them? The current trend is to use them for improving arthritic joint symptoms of pain and lack of mobility. The stems cells are injected directly into the joint or, depending on the pathology, the most severe points of tenderness around the joint. Stem cells can be stained with a radioactive dye and the most exciting thing occurs. Using X-rays, we can follow where those stem cells disappear and most of the time they hunt out and find damaged tissue to repair.

The other factor that needs to be considered is using stem cells for future insurance of one's health. If we harvest the stem cells and store them, they can potentially be used for future medical treatments against diseases many years later. So the earlier we harvest the stem cells, the less they have aged and the better likely their outcome for future use. In a sense, this is what occurs with harvesting placenta cells at the time of childbirth. My wife and I have placenta cells stored for all of our three children.

5HTP

5HTP is a natural compound found in the diet and it happens to be the precursor to serotonin; serotonin is the brain chemical that has been called the "happiness neurotransmitter". Therefore, 5HTP supplements can have an effect on improving states of depression. Quite simply, to me, 5HTP is the greatest non-pharmaceutical supplement ever invented. It saved me from having to go down the road of anti-depressants. It is my one wonder supplement that I recommend to anyone who is feeling down.

Aminoguanidine

Aminoguanidine is an extract of the herb *Goat's Rue* and it shares many similar properties with the type-II diabetic drug, *metformin*. This is interesting because both protect against the effects of diabetes, namely they improve insulin resistance and they also inhibit the very damaging effects of advanced glycated end-products (AGE), which are found at dramatically higher levels in diabetic patients. Actually, aminoguanidine has been proven to be the single best inhibitor of these damaging AGE products. AGE by-products are implicated not only in diabetes, but also in cardiovascular disease and even the development of cataracts. Since we all lose insulin sensitivity as we age, the ability to improve it can help restore day-long energy levels and ensure greater fat burning and ergo leaner body mass.

Carnosine

Carnosine is a di-peptide (two amino acids linked together) found in meats and green leafy vegetables. It is used both in top-end skin creams and in oral capsules; carnosine has many beneficial anti-ageing properties, including protection against damaging lipoproteins leading, as one example, to improved skin condition. Carnosine also blocks the effects of lactic acid in muscles which can extend sports/exercise activities. It is lactic acid that causes pain in muscles after exercise and therefore carnosine supplements reduce and delay the pain.

CoQ10

CoQ10 is a vital part of the energy systems within the body and necessary for properly functioning mitochondrial activity. It is known to be an important cardiovascular protective agent, and any patient consuming a statin drug to lower their cholesterol levels must supplement with CoQ10. A recent development is the combination of CoQ10 with a starch called cyclodextrin.

Together they increase CoQ10's bioavailability (in other words, more CoQ10 makes it into the bloodstream).

Deprenyl (see description in Smarts Drugs section below)

DHEA

DHEA is a hormone produced from the adrenal glands (situated in the kidneys), that goes on to be converted into a number of other hormones including testosterone. DHEA is the most abundant circulating sterone in blood, but as is often the case with most hormones, its production declines with advancing age. Its supplementation by men not only helps to improve testosterone levels, but in some trials it has also been shown to improve immunity. Note: I prefer the actions of the slower time-released types of DHEA.

Growth hormone

Growth hormone (GH) is a topic for a book all by itself, and indeed, I have devoted a whole chapter (4) to this key treatment in this book. For now, here is some basic background. It was in the 1980s when Dr. Daniel Rudman first proved that GH injected subcutaneously (just under the skin) was able to reverse many biological age measurements for his 60 to 70-year-old patients; in some cases lowering them by as much as 20 years. The differences noted over a three-month treatment period were better skin elasticity and thickness, improved hair density and colour, eyesight improvements, greater sense of well-being and, of course, reduced fat content and increased muscle mass, which leads to improved body shape and physical strength. However, injected recumbent human (synthetically produced) GH remains controversial, and because of its anabolic effects, it has been made a controlled substance in some countries. However, there can be little doubt about its ability to counter many of the consequences of ageing in a short period of time. Meanwhile, there are numerous agents that have been shown to improve levels of GH (without being GH themselves); for example, the amino acids arginine and glycine. In my opinion, the best non-GH agents to use include GABOB, GHRP6 and, in particular, the precursor to GH itself, sermorelin. The advantage of all these non-GH supplements is that in order to be effective, they do not have to be injected as GH itself does; in fact, these agonists can be used orally or taken sublingually (placed under the tongue).

Hydergine (see description in Smart Drugs section below)

Melatonin

Melatonin is produced by the pineal gland; a gland central to the brain and often claimed by many religions to be the "third eye". As with most hormones, melatonin levels decrease as we age. The work of Professor Walter Pierpaoli has established that melatonin has a protective effect on the pineal gland, and it ensures that the body is in control of its day-night circadian rhythms. When darkness falls, the pineal gland starts to produce melatonin. It is a physiological trigger to night, and since all hormonal cycles are based around knowing whether it is day or night, you can begin to understand the importance of melatonin. While many people know that melatonin can be a great aid in cases of jet lag, sleep disorders and shift-work pattern adherence, not many are aware of the breadth of clinical studies that have established melatonin to be efficacious in all manner of problems, including age-related macular degeneration, cancer, depression, immunity and even fertility. Fundamentally, when melatonin supplements are taken at bedtime over a few months, they stabilize circadian rhythms; this in turn stabilizes hormonal cycles and that in turn helps to stabilize immunity. Many in the field consider melatonin to be the "aspirin" of anti-ageing medicine.

Modafinil (see description under Smart Drugs section below)

Oxytocin

Oxytocin is a hormone produced by the pituitary gland in the brain. It is perhaps best known because it is given to pregnant women to help with the birth of the child, but like all hormones, oxytocin has many different uses. While there are a number of other medical uses in the literature, oxytocin is being focused on for its ability to create feelings of bonding between partners and its ability to induce a state of arousal in both men and (rather unusually) in women too. Oxytocin taken prior to sex can help to heighten the state of the orgasm in men, and has even been noted for inducing multiple orgasms in women.

Piracetam (*see description in Smart Drugs section below*)

Testosterone

Testosterone is the fundamental male hormone. Low levels of testosterone have many implications for men, including erectile dysfunction, lack of libido, muscle loss, fat gain, depression, poor sleep and general lack of "joy of life". Therefore, supplementing with testosterone can have many benefits for men. Some men use a bio-identical cream and apply it onto the inner thighs; bio-identical means it is the same molecule that is made by the testes. Since testosterone (because of its anabolic effects) has been made a controlled substance in most countries, it is something your doctor will have to help you with and you may need to obtain higher strength testosterone creams from compounding pharmacies. But there are also some useful supplements that can be used to increase testosterone levels naturally; these include tribulus terrestus, fluctoborate and zinc.

Vitamin C

Vitamin C is unique among the vitamins since it can't be stored by the human body and therefore must be captured in the diet very regularly. Twice Nobel Laureate Linus Pauling advocated high doses of vitamin C to help protect against many serious conditions, including arteriosclerosis and cancer. Vitamin C has many benefits throughout the body, but the interested reader may want to seek out a book by Dr. Thomas Levy on the subject. To take the higher doses, seek a stabilized vitamin C powder to drink in juice or water, in order to avoid stomach upset.

Vitamin D

Vitamin D could equally be a hormone as much as a vitamin. While it can be found in the diet (particularly in fish), it is principally manufactured inside the body (from cholesterol) when we expose ourselves to sunshine. Healthy vitamin D levels are essential for strong bone condition (by helping us absorb calcium) and may help protect against high blood pressure, cancer, cardiovascular disease, diabetes and autoimmune diseases.

Zinc

Zinc is a trace mineral. While it is becoming scarcer in today's soils and therefore in today's foods, it is nonetheless known to be involved in more than 300 enzymatic pathways in the body; therefore zinc is an essential element in very many processes throughout the body. For men, zinc is a crucial factor for both spermatogenesis and the production of testosterone. It therefore follows that a diet rich in zinc or regular zinc supplementation has many benefits for men.

Smart Drugs

So-called "smart drugs" have become prevalent in the anti-ageing world recently, and are considered to be the future as we harness the power to tailor drugs to individual requirements. I have tried the majority of these smart drugs with positive results.

Rather than hear any more from me on this increasingly important area of anti-ageing, I will allow an expert – Phil Micans – to give you an overview of the whole sector and the most popular smart drugs available today.

Smart Drugs and Nutrients: Their Positive Role for the Healthy Ageing Individual

By Phil Micans, MS, PharmB

I have been trained in both pharmacy and nutrition, and sometimes I feel that I can view things from a different, perhaps more holistic perspective than some of my colleagues trained in just one health profession. My case in point involves smart drugs and nutrients (herein referred to as SD). When I first became interested, dare I say fascinated, in SD in the mid-1980s, the concept seemed quite alien. Some objected to the idea of SD being used to help to counterbalance and enhance the effects of "mere" age-related mental decline.

For the objectors, it's alright to use SD to treat senile dementia or a recognized medical disorder, but their reasoning doesn't extend to improving and preventing general cognitive "issues" that (as they would argue) "naturally" occur as we age. These people believe you should put up with the memory problems that ageing brings with it; that is, until it's a really bad, medically recognized issue, and then it's alright to act! Do we treat our cars like this? Do we wait until the engine throws a camshaft and needs a major overhaul? No, we change the oil every year to make sure it doesn't ever do so, and I believe we need to apply such thinking to ageing.

Background

What are smart drugs? Medically they are called nootropics; this is a Greek word meaning "towards the mind", coined by Dr. Giurgea in the late 1960s when he was working for UCB pharmaceuticals in Belgium.

Dr. Giurgea developed the world's first nootropic SD called piracetam; it has gone on to become one of the world's bestselling agents to enhance cognitive abilities (more specific details later). The good doctor published that there were six specific categories that any nootropic should meet, as follows:

1. *They should enhance learning and memory.*
2. *They should enhance the resistance of learned behaviours/memories to conditions which tend to disrupt them.*
3. *They should protect the brain against various physical or chemical injuries.*
4. *They should increase the efficacy of the tonic cortical/subcortical control mechanisms.*
5. *They should lack the usual pharmacology of other psychotropic drugs.*
6. *They should possess very few side effects and have extremely low toxicity.*

Research into piracetam and other nootropics has progressed over the past 30 years since Dr. Giurgea's work and his original definition (as above) have been gradually amended by most researchers. Nonetheless, the nootropics SD represent a unique class, with their broad cognition enhancing, brain protecting, low toxicity and few side effect profiles.

Dr. Ward Dean's Smart Drugs and Nutrients Books

*Ward Dean, M.D., my mentor, wrote two books (*Smart Drugs and Nutrients I *and* II*) in the late 1980s. Together they really brought to light the abilities of various SD agents to enhance memory, learning, alertness and even intelligence. Despite being what Dr. Dean himself described as technical manuals for the public, they went on to sell 250,000 physical copies (pre-Internet, remember) and ignited the media with the news that students could get better grades in their exams by using them! By the way, I understand that Dr. Dean is writing a* Smart Drugs III *in 2013, so watch out for that.*

Smart Drug Examples

So now it's time to present some examples of the classic SD, to give you the "nuts and bolts" of what is being used and why they are being used. Of course, I must state that these agents need more investigation by the individual interested in them before commencement. It doesn't necessarily follow that they will all be suitable for you, nor that they can all be used in combination. As the medical field is discovering, "one size does not fit all", but it is my sincere hope that there may be information here that you will find of interest.

As a side note, many people say, "I want to improve my memory". But what is meant by "memory" exactly? For example, is your short-term memory the weakest? Is something like "where on earth are my keys?" a common problem? What about medium-term memory; where were you last week on Sunday at 5pm? Or could it be long-term memory; for example, what was the hotel's name on your holiday last year? If these questions cannot be answered relatively quickly and the problem is getting worse, then something should be done.

Perhaps your memory is okay; in other words the detail is good, but it takes a long time to recall. If so, it could be the speed of memory recall at fault rather than the memory detail by itself. And is a lack of attention, poor concentration or easy boredom to blame? If it is, how can one be expected to remember something later on with detail? If you are aware that your memory is fine for learned items of the past, but more recently learned materials are poorly remembered, then look at your attention, concentration and focus to see if memory imprinting is at fault.

Always try to recognize the weakest part of your cognition and address it.

THE AGE-NOSTIC MAN

Like any machine (even a complex human one), we are only as strong as our weakest point. Eventually, the preciseness of the investigation will lead you onto the right type of approach and enhance your cognitive abilities.

Here is an alphabetical list of more commonly used smart drugs:

Centrophenoxine (pronounced cent-row-fen-ox-in)

Centrophenoxine is a derivative of DMAE, a natural substance found principally in fish. It appears to be able to raise acetyl-l-choline, the neurotransmitter most affected in Alzheimer's disease. Furthermore, it appears to be an effective remover of the types of plagues found in that disease. Those plagues are made up of lipofuscin, a deposit that accumulates in many cells and once imbalanced can impair the cells' performance and function. In fact, centrophenoxine is recommended by Professor Imre Zs.-Nagy, a world expert in cell function and the creator of the "membrane hypothesis of ageing".

In healthy individuals, centrophenoxine appears to be an effective agent to enhance the speed of memory recall. If you want to appear sharper and more "on the ball", centrophenoxine is a good agent to consider.

Deprenyl (pronounced dep-ren-ill)

Also known as selegiline, deprenyl is a recognized treatment for Parkinson's disease because it increases the levels of the neurotransmitter most affected in that disease – dopamine. The work of Professor Joseph Knoll has shown that deprenyl supplements can help counter and improve the age-related decline of dopamine. In Professor Knoll's animal experiments, this had a very significant impact on their longevity.

In healthy humans, low doses of deprenyl (naturally, these are much less than those used for a Parkinsonian patient) exhibit effects such as improved focus and attention to detail; there is also enhanced libido/sexual desire, particularly for men, and often deprenyl can act as an anti-depressant too.

Hydergine (pronounced hi-der-gene)

Hydergine contains ergoloid mesylate, which is a fungi extract grown on rye. It has been used relatively unsuccessfully for the treatment of Alzheimer's disease (although many in the field believe that the hydergine doses have been too low for that purpose), because it has some effect on improving levels of the affected neurotransmitter acetyl-l-choline.

However, a more interesting aspect to hydergine is its ability to maintain healthy oxygen levels in the brain. Hydergine has been shown to improve oxygen levels, and in some emergency rooms around the world it is used on patients arriving from states of electrocution or drowning. This is because oxygen is a key energy element in the brain and a lack of it can very quickly lead to serious consequences; starvation of oxygen to the brain will result in death much faster than starvation of oxygen to the lungs. In healthy individuals, hydergine supplements can improve mental workload, i.e. the ability to concentrate at higher levels for longer periods before the effects of "brain fade" set in.

Modafinil (pronounced mow-daff-a-nill)

Modafinil has become a very popular "recreational" drug despite its original use being to treat narcolepsy (involuntary sleeping in the daytime). Like many revolutions in Pharma, modafinil was originally a secret agent! In this case, it was developed for the French military to allow its elite forces to remain alert and vigilant for very long periods. Importantly, there is no up or downside to modafinil; it appears to keep your attention and alertness on an even keel. It is claimed that if you are already "cognizant" it doesn't "take you higher", but if you are flagging, it "picks you up". This, coupled with its paucity of side effects, means that modafinil is no longer the domain of secret military forces; it is now used by pilots, air traffic controllers, surgeons, stock exchange traders and truck drivers, etc. to help them maintain their abilities at a high level.

Piracetam (pronounced pie-rass-i-tam)

Piracetam, as was mentioned in my introduction, is the original SD created by "cleaving" it from GABA, a natural agent found in the diet. Originally, piracetam was approved for treating travel and altitude sickness, but shortly afterward it was discovered to help people be creative and improve their short-term memory status. Piracetam operates by improving electrical communication across the corpus callosum (the central part of the brain; the bit that holds the two hemispheres together). Some believe that the corpus callosum can sometimes act as a "road block" as it tries to pass electrical information from one side of the brain to the other.

Healthy persons using piracetam appear to improve their short-term memory and have a heightened state of awareness. Perhaps unsurprisingly, because of its previously described actions, it appears to promote ingenuity and the ability to see these ideas into design.

Vasopressin (pronounced vase-o-press-in)

Vasopressin is actually a peptide hormone found in the brain's hippocampus, where it is believed to be responsible for "laying down" memories. Usually taken as a nasal spray, its approved use is to help prevent frequent urination, and it is often prescribed to men with prostate problems who otherwise would be running to the toilet during the night. But vasopressin's less well-known role is in aiding memory, and it has even been applied in states of amnesia.

For healthy individuals, the role of vasopressin is interesting since it is a significant imprinter. That is to say, vasopressin is not very likely to help with already learned memories, but it will be able to assist in memories yet to be learned. Vasopressin nasal sprays are usually of porcine origin, whereas the synthetic version is referred to as desmopressin.

Conclusion

There are not only stacks of anecdotal evidence that SD can improve an individual's cognitive performance, self-evident by their popularity among students to improve their exam results, but there is also mounting published clinical evidence of their efficacy. For example, a clinical trial conducted by Dr. Dimond and Dr. Brouwers reported on the results of some of a series of seven double-blind trials. They involved 16 second and third-year college students who were in excellent health and good physical and mental condition. The subjects received either 4,800mg a day of piracetam or a placebo (a non-active substance) for 14 days. In three different measures of verbal learning and memory, the results showed a highly significant difference in favour of the piracetam students over the placebo controls.

In the authors' conclusion, they stated: "The fact is that piracetam improves verbal learning and in this it would appear to be a substance which is capable of extending the intellectual functions of man. Our subjects were not senile, nor suffering from generalized brain disorder, confusional states or any other pathology of the brain. It is therefore possible to extend the power which [individuals already gifted with high intelligence and good memory] possess to still higher levels despite the fact that the range of their achievement is already high."

Ten tips for embarking upon the anti-ageing journey:

1. You will hear and read conflicting opinions.
2. Do your own research.
3. Feel and see the results.
4. You will take at least 10 years off.
5. Don't listen to traditional views and beliefs about ageing.
6. You are not your father.
7. Anti-ageing technology and treatments are only getting more advanced.
8. It's never too late to start.
9. It's OK to be different.
10. Remain excited about the journey.

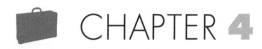

CHAPTER 4

SO, WHERE DO I GET IT?

The power of hormone replacement therapy

One of the main cornerstones of age-nostic medicine is hormone replacement, and specifically HGH or human growth hormone. The scientist that came up with the term "human growth hormone" was clearly not a marketer as the name is hardly comforting, conjuring up all types of thoughts. Combining this with the many different opinions on the Internet, one could automatically be very hesitant about trying such a product, just as I was at first. The fact that injecting growth hormone is the most effective way of taking it further makes one think this is not a path worth taking.

The information about side effects, in my opinion, is very misguided and often extreme. The fact that you can find information that says taking growth hormone will cause your hands and feet to swell and cause pain in the joints is scary at the very least. This is similar to reading an American magazine that is advertising a particular drug; it contains an abundance of warnings and possible side effects. Its aim seems to be to get you to think that taking any particular drug on the market will cause horrendous harm and possibly lead to death in nearly all cases. The list of possible and potentially dangerous side effects is so extreme that the average consumer ends up living in constant fear regardless of what they are taking. Either that, or we choose to ignore them. These types of warnings are political correctness gone completely mad: would we have half the life-saving medical treatments we have now if everyone took this attitude when something new is discovered?

Like most things in age-nostic medicine, it is all about the dosage. Taking a safe amount – like a small glass of vodka rather than a bottle, like a single meal of junk food rather than one every day – is the key. I have never had any side effects whatsoever from taking hormone replacement treatments or from any other parts of the age-nostic lifestyle. By taking treatments in the correct dosage and "listening" to what my body has to say every step of the way, I have only had the benefits of such treatments.

A Background to HGH

HGH is the first substance to have been clinically proven to reverse the effects of ageing, having been validated by a number of rigorous double-blind, placebo-controlled clinical studies. The ground-breaking work of Dr. Daniel Rudman published in the highly respected *New England Journal of Medicine* in 1990 marked the beginning of the use of HGH as an anti-ageing medicine.

Dr. Rudman undertook a six-month trial of HGH supplementation in 12 men aged from 61 to 81. Every single one of the study participants gained muscle and bone density, lost fat, thickened their skin and expanded their livers and spleens after taking HGH. What makes these results even more astonishing is that all of these positive changes were achieved without the participants altering their diets, lifestyles or smoking habits. Dr. Rudman concluded that the HGH supplementation regime he had placed the men on had, in effect, reversed their biological age by 10 to 20 years! Dr. Rudman's remarkable results have since been verified by further clinical trials which have also demonstrated the safety and effectiveness of HGH supplementation.

The benefits of using HGH therapy include:

- Loss of body fat leading to significant weight loss. For example, in Dr. Rudman's study, the men lost on average 14% of their body fat.
- Increased lean muscle mass. Again, in Dr. Rudman's study, the men gained on average 8.8% lean muscle mass. This results in increased strength. HGH therapy has also been used to counteract the effects of muscle wasting in AIDS patients.
- Improvements in skin thickness and elasticity. This can manifest itself as a reduction in wrinkles and the re-appearance of a more youthful skin tone.
- Enhanced feelings of general well-being and a reduction in feelings of depression and anxiety, along with improved emotional stability and a more optimistic outlook.
- Strengthening of the immune system. Our immune systems become much less effective as we age, making us prone to the development of a

whole raft of diseases. By strengthening our immune systems, not only are we less susceptible to infection and disease, but recovery from illness is aided and immune-related diseases become less troublesome for us. Allergies also improve.

- Increased sexual potency and libido.
- Increased energy levels and vitality with improved stamina.
- Improved sleeping patterns with better quality sleep.
- Improved digestion.
- Improved mental processes.
- Improved nail growth and hair condition.
- Increased LDL cholesterol (the "good" cholesterol).
- Improved eyesight.

It's Controversial!

As I stated earlier, many of the treatments and therapies mentioned in this book are relatively new, and therefore, the more conservative amongst the medical fraternity are wary and indeed quite openly hostile towards them. This has been the case for HGH, testosterone and other hormone replacement therapies.

My good friend and contributor to this book, Dr. Michael Zacharia, who, despite never having prescribed any illegal medication, was brought before a tribunal hearing looking into his prescriptions of HGH, testosterone and other testosterone-promoting medications to a small number of patients. In the end, it was ruled that he should not prescribe HGH, testosterone or anabolic steroids. He also had to complete an ethics course. Two years after this event, the prescription of these substances is practiced widely throughout the world, and in fact there is more evidence now to suggest that the use of testosterone and HGH is indicated in certain patients for hormone replacement therapy and also in anti-ageing medicine. Yet, Dr. Zacharia is still not allowed to prescribe any of these hormones or practice anti-ageing medicine. He continues to practice his other areas of medicine and surgery and all his patients requesting anti-ageing assessments are referred to and managed by fellow medical practitioners.

The discovery of new medicines and treatments tend to go through a long period of testing before being accepted by the medical establishment. Nevertheless, in the case of anti-ageing treatments like hormone replacement, this has not stopped their usage increasing quite dramatically over recent years, even if they have not yet gained wide recognition from the medical fraternity. There are many articles today about the life-saving potential of certain cancer treatments that have been years in trial or are simply not economical enough for companies to do the long-term research and development required to get them approved for public usage. Unfortunately for cancer patients, attaining the benefits of such treatments has been much less easier. The reality is certain medicines and treatments which have not undergone long-term testing will still find their way into the marketplace simply because evidence and research shows that they do work and people want them. This has certainly been the case for many of the anti-ageing medicines and treatments described in this book.

Testosterone is another important hormone for men and testosterone replacement therapy is widely accepted in the United States. In fact, the treatment is regularly promoted and advertised through mainstream TV. However, in the UK and other countries, you won't see such promotions and advertisements. That each country has a different view or rule further adds to the confusion for people on the real truth and benefits of hormone replacement treatments and therapies.

Many of today's anti-ageing treatments, including hormone replacement, originated in the body-building industry and gradually filtered out to the wider public. The link with sports doping and performance enhancement often creates a wrong impression about hormone replacement. Those professional sports people who are caught using performance-enhancing drugs cause near hysteria amongst sports authorities and fellow athletes – and quite rightly so. But for the average man, who has access to such treatments, why shouldn't they enhance their performance, health and general well-being? As we age, these vital hormones begin to decline. But there are treatments and supplements available for men to replace these lost hormones and help them to manage the ageing process in a positive way. For example, growth hormones are essential to keep our organs in good shape. If our organs are in bad shape, we are going to have a pretty tough time of it. So, given the choice, why wouldn't any man want to consider hormone replacement treatments and supplements?

The message that men do have choices and options in the whole ageing process is one that I am passionate about broadcasting, and this book is the beginning of that. Here, I have simply outlined my own experience in making these choices and using anti-ageing medicines, including any side effects (which have largely been absent in my case). Finding and working with good medical doctors, who can conduct the correct tests and provide sensible treatments, is of course something that I would highly recommend to all of you when it comes to hormone replacement therapy and indeed in your entire age-nostic journey. The body is a complex thing and you often have to assess a number of factors before deciding upon a particular treatment or supplement. Saying that, it is quite a challenge to find a medical doctor willing to go on the record about anti-ageing treatments, even if there are numerous doctors prescribing such treatments. Like most things in life, the majority of professionals will be responsible and conduct the necessary tests and prescribe the right treatments, but there will always be a few medical practitioners who will not do so.

Most people, when they start to consider hormone replacement therapy, will do their own research via the Internet. By doing that, you will usually come across totally conflicting viewpoints, warnings and opinions. You will come across sites openly advertising hormone replacement therapies and supplements. Never buy such products via the Internet. Most of the time, you will not be able to confirm the source or legitimacy of what you are buying. A black market has already opened up for HGH. Again, you cannot be sure of its origins and legitimacy. Yes, you should do your own research and learn as much as you can about hormone replacement, but then find a good medical doctor/clinic that specializes in anti-ageing treatments, who/which can do the correct tests on you, and then prescribe the right treatment.

For me, quality of life is what I am really interested in, and in particular, the longevity part of it. As I research more and see what is coming in the years ahead, I believe growth hormone and many other treatments are like the first cars or electronic products which appeared – in other words, anti-ageing medicines are still in their infancy today, but these treatments will advance and grow exponentially, and the benefits of these new treatments will be so exciting for men.

Hormone replacement therapy is, of course, not for everyone – at least for now. Like most relatively new things that come on to the market, it takes pioneers to experiment and judge the benefits. I am one of these pioneers. To end this chapter, here's the story of another pioneer who embraced hormone replacement therapy and the age-nostic lifestyle in general. He is a colleague and friend and he actually wrote this letter to me after his transition to age-nostic man.

Hey Michael,

There are no other words for it other than to say you have changed my life for the better in so many ways. Thank you.

Late last year things started to change. I was feeling more tired, falling asleep on the couch at night after five minutes, waking up a bit muzzy and a few weird things were starting to happen.

I was losing some of my core strength – very hard to explain, but as a man you notice if this kind of thing changes, even a small amount. I was also losing a bit of my memory which for me was frightening. And my desire for sex was dwindling rapidly – a happy, healthy two to three times a week (not bad after 18 years of marriage) was lucky to be once a month. And when we did do what married couples do, my performance was about as impressive as the England World Cup team in South Africa.

Even scoring a goal didn't feel like it used to (shock horror for a red blooded male – why else are we alive I kept thinking?).

Being married to a sensual, beautiful half-Polish, half-Dutch woman, whose expectations are greater than Manchester United fans, I was really starting to get worried.

Then – and I still can't explain it – I started to go down a slippery slope – fast! My work, which is my life blood, wasn't that attractive anymore. I was lacking energy, my ambitions were changing, my relationship with my wife was tense and for the first time ever I was starting to think that my time was up early and that I had better jump out of corporate life and think about the next 20 years.

Perhaps the most bewildering was the fact I was getting emotional – I was welling up on a regular basis – very weird for a man in the prime of his life. The movie Marley and Me *was traumatic for me! I even had to leave the room when a couple of favourites were voted out of* The X-Factor.

Seriously, random bouts of emotion and tears just made the situation even more distressing and worrisome.

Conscious of burn-out, stress-led heart attacks and the like across many of my peers, I started to plan my exit – I want to meet my grandchildren and hopefully my great grandchildren, so being one for prevention rather than cure, I started to put the plan in motion.

However, this constant nagging doubt was in my head that I wasn't ready and that I had so much more to give, plus I knew so many guys much older than me with so much energy, spark and who didn't seem to be having a lot of trouble in the horizontal jogging department.

So why me?

The other thing that is not taken into consideration in all of this is that the good old male ego takes a bashing and you can't explain the embarrassment and shame you start to feel when "shit" you can't explain starts to "happen" to you. "I am only 42 for heaven's sake," I kept saying to myself a little less eloquently.

So what does one do in the naughties?

Phone a friend and good old Google – one day God is going to make an appearance and admit he/she is the man/woman behind Google.

You were great and you told me to jump on Google and find a doctor who tested for testosterone levels.

I had never had an "MOT for a man" before and must say I will never forget the fear when I heard those rubber gloves snap and I was told to roll over; and I will never forget the relief when I was told things were normal in the big "p" department.

So Mr. Sceptical then proceeds to sit down and after many questions to the doctor I now realize in hindsight this was the moment in my life that I will look

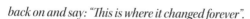

back on and say: "This is where it changed forever".

I was told I should work on my cholesterol and blood sugar and I should lose a bit of weight, but my blood pressure was fine and I was doing what I do without any track record of sickness (my last genuine sick day was four years ago). In short, I was a typical 42-year-old.

EXCEPT my testosterone was at a low level. All I remember was that I should have had a score in the 20s but I was 8.5 – and I remember a little burst of adrenalin kicking in. This is what I will now reflect on as the burst of "hope adrenalin" – could this be the answer? What if I could get my levels into the 20s – would I, could I, will I be able to get out of this nightmare that was plaguing me?

I half listened to what the doc was telling me about getting results with quite a few men and that testosterone replacement therapy could also help me. The rest was a blur. I remember the practice manager giving me a box of gel and that I had to rub it on my bare shoulders every morning and come back in three months.

Off I went with a degree of hope, optimism and, I have to say, a little desperation.

Over the next week things began to change as I religiously applied my gel each morning. Gradually, there was an increase in my strength, I could feel my alertness returning, my memory was sharper and low and behold there was a bit of movement below the belt...four weeks into the treatment and I am a different man – a lot more energy, work is a breeze. Even leading a global rebranding project across 10 companies and 26 countries became an exciting challenge I was looking forward to tackling every day rather than seeing it as the end of the world.

My libido was returning to some kind of normality and my wife was looking at me the way she used to – which I cannot tell you what a relief this is given where I had spiralled to.

Eight weeks into the treatment and I can honestly say I felt like a new man – my strength was back, my manliness was back, I had energy, my ambition had been restored, my passion, my desire and my zest for life and everything I love in it was special again. And when you are running a global company I think it goes without saying what it means to be not only back to normal but improving on normal. Every week I was improving.

12 weeks in and the strength is building – I could feel my muscles getting harder – literally. My horizontal jogging had gone to the next level even to the point where we both feel like honeymooners again and can honestly say I feel so much healthier, happier and alert.

What had been exciting me even more was that I knew there was more in there (if that makes sense) – there is another level and I was praying as I was coming in for my re-assessment that there would be a way to increase this phenomenal path I was on.

So to the re-assessment – thank god the doctor didn't move towards the rubber glove cupboard again.

I was genuinely nervous to see what had transpired over three months on the technical side of things.

My results = wow!

- I had lost weight.
- My cholesterol had reduced.
- My blood sugar had reduced.
- My blood pressure had improved from the first session.
- And my testosterone had gone from 8.5 to 14.1!

So given I need to be in the 20s to tick the box, I cannot tell you how excited I was at the prospect of improving my health and lifestyle to what is effectively a tripling from where I started – the change from 8.5 to 14 has been incredible and I could not wait to keep improving.

Thank God I made that call, Michael, and I thank you from every fibre of my being for rescuing me from sliding down a slippery slope to feeling amazing – it is hard to explain the difference from where I was to where I am now. It is unbelievable.

I also hope my story helps other men to put their pride aside (and fear of the snapping of those rubber gloves) and take the leap of faith to test themselves.

Feel free to share my experience with whomever you want – it is real and it is absolutely incredible what has happened to me!

Get a Good Night's Sleep

Thousands and thousands of men over 40 suffer from sleep deprivation of one sort or another, and this will definitely affect the production of critical hormones. Men who are chronic snorers think they are having a good night's sleep, but when they wake up, they feel tired and unrefreshed. The same goes for the unfortunate partners who have to share their beds! Indeed, so many relationships turn sour because men are snoring and don't (or won't) do anything about it.

60% of men over 40 are chronic snorers and have a sleep apnea. If not treated, it can be a silent killer. Your brain and vital organs are literally starved of oxygen, because you stop breathing as a result of your airways being blocked while snoring. To be deprived of this amount of oxygen night after night is incredibly unhealthy and many diseases form in our sleep as a result. Moreover, sleep apnea and other issues that cause sleep deprivation will affect the production of key hormones. There is a huge amount of research which demonstrates sleep's contribution to our hormone production, energy levels, our moods and overall health.

So, for all you men who aren't sleeping well or are snoring like a Harley Davidson, get yourselves to a sleep clinic or specialist. A friend of mine did exactly this. By that point, he was sleeping in the spare room after being kicked out of the marital bed. He was invited to take a simple sleep test by the specialist. The test showed he had stopped breathing 38 times an hour in a seven-hour sleep cycle, with 10 instances where he had given up breathing for more than a minute! The specialist advised it was a very scary scenario and something that had to be sorted out - and fast! Through the use of a mouth guard, his snoring has been cured and his life has changed completely. He is waking up refreshed, his blood pressure has reduced, his blood sugars have returned from high to normal, his cholesterol level is down significantly and his overall health has improved dramatically. Most importantly, he is back in the marital bed.

Dr. Aditi Desai, a leading Harley Street dentist with a special interest in dental sleep medicine (and a Honorary Research Fellow at the Sleep

Disorders Unit at King's College London), said: "Sleep is the most essential part of a person's well-being and any level of sleep deprivation leads to a metabolic chain of events with serious health consequences." So, bite the bullet and get tested if you are a snorer. Even if you are not a snorer but wake up tired most days, the test will reveal why you are sleeping badly. A sleep test and the resulting treatment could not only help you improve your hormone production and general well-being, it could more importantly save your life.

Ten tips for considering and having hormone replacement treatment:
1. Get a full blood test first to check your hormone levels.
2. Research as much as possible and keep an open mind.
3. Don't start before 40 years of age unless your blood test shows significant deficiency.
4. Get regular blood tests (every three months) to test your levels.
5. Monitor the benefits.
6. Be realistic.
7. Be patient – it could take three to six months to see significant change.
8. Don't get spooked by negative scare-mongering.
9. Only order from a licensed medical source.
10. Take regular breaks and monitor the changes.

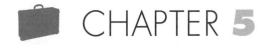

CHAPTER 5

THE MID-LIFE CRISIS

Why it's happening to so many men

What a strange term "mid-life crisis" is! Since this predicament often seems to happen in our 40s or early 50s, it assumes we are all going to live till 90 or 100 years. The fact is, this metamorphosis usually occurs at a period in our life when we suddenly feel that more time has passed in our lives than we believe is left. One of the main factors in stimulating this event is that our own role models – often our fathers – are starting to show us that the future may not be as good as we had thought. We watch our parents age, often rapidly, and in many cases pass away from diseases such as cancer, and we are reminded of our own mortality. I know in my own case that watching my father decline and literally give up had a huge effect on me. It was a hugely negative experience and affected more parts of my life than I thought was possible.

There is no coincidence that the majority of marriage breakdowns happen in this very same period of our lives. If you have started a family at the usual time, your children are often coming to maturity and in many cases leaving home as we reach a critical time in our own life. This can put additional pressure on the relationship, especially for the woman who has spent the best part of her life doing the majority of the parenting. A huge hole is created in a woman's life, and what had been the glue that bound her life together for many years can suddenly become unstuck. It can expose real flaws in most relationships. A family unit with all the diversions suddenly becomes a two-person partnership and the dynamics affect everyone.

I started to question all facets of my life in my mid-40s. Was my marriage really as good as I thought it was? Was my career what really made me happy? Was I financially in the position to change direction or was this also too late? I had made so many changes in my 30s, but could always bounce back quickly because so many good years were still ahead. Was this the case as I approached my 50th birthday? Society had drilled into me, like most other men, that the future was about wind down, slow down, followed by break down. There were so many unhappy marriages around and lots of disorientated people. I spoke to many senior business people about their frustrations with their careers, and in too many cases there was simply a resignation that it was too late to change, too late to save what was once a happy marriage or stellar career.

In London, where I spend time, the media is full of advertisements warning us of the precarious position someone over 50 years of age finds themselves in. If we have not planned for our financial future, we are brainwashed into believing that after 50 it is a downhill slope towards a nursing home. I was shocked recently to watch an ad from a well-known insurance firm, which was for over 50s offering a seniors discount. It was as if I was already in need of urgent medical assistance of some kind. I still felt young, yet others believed I was already old and way over the hill.

Also, the media constantly bombards us with images of famous and successful men with beautiful young women by their side, often 20 years younger than themselves, living what is perceived as an ideal lifestyle. The world around us is full of stories of men leaving their marriages to start up with someone much younger in the hope that this one thing will roll back the clock. It will not unless you have an age-nostic outlook on life and manage to live and feel as if you are much younger. I have dated girls in the past few years who are much younger than me but never for that reason. I do, however, enjoy the youthful energy that such relationships bring, along with the obvious feeling that I am capable of living an energetic life.

If you are not in a relationship at the moment or have never settled down, it is possible that the same feelings of panic and resignation can occur. In most cases, your energy has been put into your career and you are suddenly faced with the thought of having possibly missed the boat. There is also the nagging doubt as to whether you will ever find anyone at this stage in your life. If you are not in a brilliant financial situation, the sense of resignation can hang around for some time. And as a result of constant media images, there is a feeling that only the wealthy guys get the beautiful younger women.

The reason for partnerships between older men and younger women is a very controversial subject. Many women will think that the girl is with the man because he is wealthy. All I can say is that in the two serious relationships I have had since my divorce, this was not the case. I was not rich and was still striving to rebuild my wealth. I believe what attracted the girls was my enthusiasm, appetite for life and age-nostic outlook. This instilled a feeling of security, which is an important part of women's natural, often unconscious, need.

Divorce and Break-up

This is a particularly hard thing to write about because I regret my own divorce very much. However, a book about men and what happens as we get older would be a little pointless without some commentary on this and the damage it causes to all those involved.

If you get married in your early 30s, it is similar to a career choice. Often it is not necessarily well thought out. Suddenly an opportunity comes up and it looks like it is what we want. Two people are in the zone to start a life together and suddenly, before you know it, you are married, having a family, and life takes on a momentum all of its own. The test only really comes later in life as you both reach crossroads and the changes that brings into the relationship.

I met and married a beautiful girl who was everything I was not. How often does that happen to us men? My ex-wife was elegant, beautiful, calm, pragmatic and very understanding. She was loyal to the end. When I met her, it was love at first sight. It remained that way for the entire marriage.

She came from a Hungarian immigrant family who had escaped across the border to Austria in the middle of the night, already with one small child. My mother-in-law had been brought up with the best private schooling in Budapest and got married at a young age to the man she loved. He was a tall, incredibly handsome country boy who loved hunting and spending his time in the forest.

They needed to leave Hungary quickly because her father was about to be arrested. Many were, for no apparent reason in those times. I can only imagine what it must have been like to leave everything behind for an unknown place. Once they had escaped, they ended up in a refugee camp with virtually nothing. The choice was Canada or Australia, and they very much wanted to go to Canada. However, they arrived in the most remote place in the world, Perth, and at the hottest time of the year. They worked hard and made a life having three more children, my ex-wife being the last.

Fast forward 30 years, and my ex-wife meets a blue-eyed, blond New Zealander, who talks far too fast and has far too grand plans. Later, I hope the energy and enthusiasm I had at 30 was what attracted her to me. For months she wouldn't show much interest, but I continued to pursue her anyway. I was really in love with this quiet beauty from such a completely different background.

It's only now that I think how difficult it must have been for her to try and understand someone like me. I had no real career plans, no money and no prospects, but I did have enthusiasm. She had built a successful career in film and television as a make-up artist and had already worked hard to buy her own small terraced house in Perth. Life was good in Perth and she was happy to have travelled since the age of 17 all over the world, back-packing through countries that even today many would not dare visit. She was not only beautiful but also worldly and wise.

Somehow I managed to move in with her after finally surviving a long courtship of her doubts. I think she tried her best to avoid showing any serious interest in me, but I persevered and, hopefully looking back, she did actually fall for me. But you never quite knew: her European background meant she never really revealed her feelings. Looking back, it was an elegant, calm kind of love that she showed.

My manic energy, and the ups and downs that this produced, was already causing some problems. It was hard for her to see a future and so she decided to go off to New York to do an advance course in make-up. At the same time, she kindly said to me that it would be best if I moved out while she was away. She wasn't harsh, she had simply decided that I was too much to handle. As always, she said it with dignity and little emotion; that was just the way she was and what I had fallen in love with.

I was suddenly alone in her house and (always the salesman) already trying to come up with a plan to present to her. I was truly in love and I needed to convince her that there was more to me.

I didn't move out and a month later she returned. As she came through the front door, she saw me sitting at the dinner table looking a bit sheepish but smiling. I jumped up, ran towards her and hugged her. She suddenly burst into tears and I was taken aback immediately. I should have left as I had promised and I felt terribly guilty. All I could think of saying was "What's wrong?", and she burst into tears with such emotion, then said, "I am pregnant."

With excitement and a huge smile on my face, I said, "Great, we can get married!" She looked even more horrified at my simple solution, as clearly I had put no thought into it. Today that is our beautiful older daughter who is now 24; we had another equally beautiful daughter who is now 19.

She supported me totally for the next 18 years without complaint, going through my constant job changes and drinking bouts, caused by my manic depression I periodically experienced, and even lent me the money to buy into my first successful business. She went through the emotional breakdown I experienced after my adventure in the Philippines.

So why does a man suddenly leave his partner and family after all this and never return? Why would any man give up so much? Like most men, I have no clear answer to this. You would think divorce should be avoided at all costs, but the statistics prove that the majority of marriage breakdowns are instigated by men during their mid-life. It is clear that breaking up a marriage can cause huge destruction for everyone involved. This is especially so for the woman who has already given up so much to support her partner and basically has spent the best part of her life bringing up children, only now to find herself alone and frightened. Women rarely leave, whereas men hit an age, begin to doubt themselves, and then often leave their partners for no real reason at all, just as I did.

Divorce is worse than experiencing a death. They say death is final and you can move on, but a divorce leaves people devastated, lost, confused and guilty. Moreover, children who basically had a solid foundation are left even more confused and hurt, no matter what age they are. The financial devastation for both parties is also profound: you have to split things up and fight over a new uncertain future. For women, divorce usually happens at the worst time in their lives, because the perception is that men tend to meet another partner quickly, usually younger, whereas no matter how beautiful a woman is later in life, it is simply so much harder for her. It really isn't fair.

Society and the law turns divorce into a painful and disorientating experience where no one wins, whatever the financial outcome. In America today, it is considered the most devastating financial experience for all parties, only slightly ahead of bankruptcy. If everyone really knew what that journey might bring, we would really think more about the whole thing.

Five years after our divorce and we are strangers and rarely talk. There is too much pain for that on both sides. Today at 53, I have learned so much and know so little. I would love to be friends with my ex-wife and for both of us to be at our daughters' weddings as a family. Maybe this book will allow us both to heal and become the friends we were for so long.

And as an age-nostic man, with the enthusiasm and energy I had when I was 30, I believe I may get another chance and meet someone as well and do it all again – but of course differently in many ways. However, having admitted all my flaws and imperfections during this journey, I may well scare off a lot of women. Nevertheless, I remain as always positive and excited about life and love, and maybe some girl will see I am just a boy who wants to fall in love with a girl. That never changes with age, no matter how old you are. And just for the record, I believe totally in marriage and would love one day to do it again.

Financial Problems

There is no worse feeling than getting to your late 40s or early 50s and realizing your finances are not where they should be. I still think most men believe they are the financial provider and bread-winner in a relationship, and things really haven't changed that much on that front for some time. I know so many people who because of their entrepreneurial nature have rebuilt their careers and finances, which gave me great hope. The pain they experienced from their initial loss drove them on, which is an admirable and much under-valued quality.

The world is full of stories of businessmen who have made a second fortune or created new wealth and financial stability. Unfortunately, most men are fearful of failure and are simply afraid to try again or change a career and end up going into shutdown/protection mode. We are conditioned to think this way, and it is actually a self-fulfilling prophecy for a sad and unfulfilling later life. Remember, if you are in such a position, you have already partially failed, but it will only be a real failure if you don't have the courage to start again. I am more excited today about starting up my new gen-agenostic health clinics business for men than any other business I have been involved in. I am so driven to have success at this stage of my life and show others that it can be done, that I am sure it will be financially more successful than I ever imagined.

Health and Rejuvenation

We have all heard of the saying "nothing else really matters except your health" and when you think about it, it is so true. I recently lost one of my closest friends to a sudden heart attack, and it really made me think about the vulnerability of life and how we must live as if there is no defined time left. He was very fit and only 46 years old with two young children, having married for the first time when he was in his early 40s. He was starting up a mining company in Brazil and had just moved his young family to Rio de Janeiro. He was running on the beach one day and had a massive heart attack, having not realized there may have been a problem. In our anti-ageing clinics, we believe in a lot of testing for all our major organs including work on genetics to warn clients of any potential undiagnosed problems.

I think of him often and it drives me on to keep remembering to enjoy every day and live as full a life as possible. It showed me that life is so unpredictable and uncertain, so live it positively and don't focus on getting older but on feeling younger. I think the biggest factor in the age-nostic lifestyle revolves around rejuvenation and repair just as much as about prevention and rolling back the clock.

While you may not want to follow the regime in this book as pathologically as I do, there are some key factors you could follow to give yourself the best chance of not following others into premature old age and suffering the dreaded mid-life crisis:

1. Accept that you are in bad shape (if that is the case) and may have prematurely aged. I am amazed at how many men I meet who are in terrible shape in their late 30s and early 40s let alone in their 50s.

2. You can't do anything without being in good mental health. If you are suffering from depression, accept it and get your mind back in a positive condition. As I still suffer from bouts of depression, I quickly change my regime by increasing supplement intake, stepping up my exercises and improving my diet further until the period has passed. Be aware that this might be the time when you will be tempted to increase self-medication (such as excessive alcohol consumption and unhealthy food intake). This will only make things worse.

3. Get fitter and more flexible by exercising and start improving your appearance.

4. Seek advice and create an action plan for change.

5. Nip any slide in health in the bud quickly. You need to start looking and feeling younger plus acting younger. This will improve all your personal relationships, especially your intimate ones.

6. We all end up in the ground, and even an age-nostic lifestyle can't change that. It should never be the fear of death that really drives you. The fear of a slow debilitating ageing process is what should frighten the hell out of you.

7. It is simply never too late to make changes. I am used to massive and rapid turns in my life, but while it can often be painful at the time, I can honestly say a better outcome has occurred.

8. Be very aware that any addiction you may have developed is now getting well advanced because of the passage of time. If you can't stop, just try and cut down because things will get worse as you get older. For example, what you could drink in terms of alcohol in your 20s and 30s and feel okay will be having a much greater effect in your 40s and 50s. This is the same with drugs and other addictive substances.

9. Watch what you eat as your metabolism has slowed and you will simply get fatter quicker. It will become harder to turn things around the older you get.

10. Visit a nursing home or hospital for the elderly. You will be shocked at how bad ageing can be from many self-induced habits. Not everyone is Steve Jobs and dies suddenly of a rare cancer; most age-related illnesses are self-induced and can be avoided.

In summary, there does not have to be a mid-life crisis, but you will probably experience one of some kind. It is possible to manage the impact on your life and the people around you. You can get through it and come out the other end a better, wiser person in the process. Dr. Michael Zacharia now provides an inspiring story to illustrate this.

Mid-Life Crisis
By Dr. Michael Zacharia

In the field of cosmetic surgery, I am always exposed to patients who seem to have their lives well and truly together but are, in fact, in the depths of a mid-life crisis. If I had to perform a psychological assessment on my patients before surgery, I probably wouldn't be operating that much! What is interesting is that both men and women suffer this crisis but respond in a varied manner. It is not only patients but also friends I have observed going through these dramatic changes in their life.

Tom is a case in point. Tom is the age-nostic man. He is good-looking, fit and healthy and has a body typical of a 30-year-old. He is ripped with a six-pack most cannot achieve in youth. Tom is 57 years old and has been through a typical mid-life period that has seen his world turn upside down. He got through it by grit and determination, but not without the greatest upheaval in his life. Now he is on the road to success once again.

I have known Tom and his family all my life. His brother and my cousin were mates and we all spent time together around my grandmother's house in Adelaide. When I moved to the Northern Territory in 1997, I was told to visit the "best restaurant in Darwin" which Tom owned. It was on the waterfront in the new marina called Cullen Bay and was by far and away the busiest and most favoured dining spot in the New Territory. Tom had a very successful video business in Adelaide, but after years of raking in copious amounts of cash, the industry crashed and he was without a business or income. He moved his wife and three boys to Darwin in the early 90s in search of a new life, and with his business partner essentially developed the multi-million dollar marina complex in Cullen Bay.

It was considered a high-risk venture because Cullen Bay was built on reclaimed land, only having been done before in Darwin. Of course, Hong Kong's new airport is built on the same platform and many others since. The development, the restaurant and the move to Darwin turned out to be a huge success. Having lost everything in his 30s and gaining it back in his 40s, life was looking good. The restaurant was hugely successful, won all sorts of awards, and was being run by Tom and all the family. But in the early part of 2000, the sands started shifting. Tom's marriage became strained, a separation ensued and all the assets he had built in Darwin fell precariously in danger as a result of being robbed by his book-keeper. Life was great and then it was bust. He lost his marriage, he was pressured into selling everything, and then in his early 50s he had nothing. Nothing!

At this point, most people might throw in the towel. And for a while so did Tom. He couldn't because he had worked hard and lost it all on two occasions. However, what he did have was support from his family (including his wife with whom he is still friends and shares his house when she is in Darwin), a fantastic attitude and an age-nostic lifestyle. He took a break for a while, maintained and improved his fitness, commenced supplements including multivitamins, zinc and the age-nostic diet, and over the next few years started looking for a new venture. And he found it. Tom researched the needs of Darwin, identified the lack of a good pizza shop in the city, worked out he could run it with his family from 5pm to 10pm. He travelled Australia to determine the best fit-out and recipes, and has now opened his new venture in the middle of Darwin in an old lingerie shop! People said he could not do it, but he has and a good reputation has made City Pizza one of the best I have been to. My own age-nostic diet includes a reduction in overall carbohydrate, but the occasional breakout for one of those wonderful pizzas is worth it on every occasion. Well done Tom, another crisis overcome.

Work-Life Balance

I have seen many mid-life crises come on as a result of work-life balance – or to be more accurate, a lack of work-life balance. The reality for many men is work and nothing besides. I predict we will see far more problems in society as the issues of work-life balance flare up further. These will include greater levels of stress, anxiety and worry about day-to-day things. A large part of the cause is down to both technology and corporate culture.

In terms of technology, which was supposed to make our lives easier, it has also made us contactable all the time. I asked a few friends recently how many take work calls or emails over the weekend and on holiday. The results – virtually all of them all the time – will not surprise many. On the culture side, many companies seem to expect employees at all levels to be contactable and work harder than they have ever done before. It seems no longer good enough to do a good job in normal working hours. This trend will not reverse unless each of us puts a marker in the sand. If we don't, the next mid-life crisis people talk about could be very close to home. Here is an interesting case in point. Paul Sanderson, a full-on CEO, provides us below with an insight into the corporate fast-lane, and how he copes with it.

"How Do You Do It?"
By Paul Sanderson, CEO

People regularly ask me, "How do you do it – how do you what you do, Paul?" We are all incredibly busy in our own way, I hear myself often say, but when Michael Hogg asked me for my take on work-life balance, I took stock of my last 12 months.

Let me first set the scene. I run a billion-dollar company; we operate in 26 countries and have around 12 active group companies. The largest of these has over 40 major clients and 800 offices. I have 14 direct reports who range from company CEOs to country COOs. We are in every time zone and my phone, texts and emails literally go 24 hours a day. A typical day starts at 7am when I get in the car with a call to KL, Moscow or Sydney and ends with contact from Canada and the US somewhere between 7-10pm. There is no time for breaks during the day and I wouldn't eat if our wonderful support team didn't feed and water me at various points of the day.

We move from meeting to meeting – one could be a board meeting; the next a presentation to the bank; a legal case in Brazil; a new product development initiative; crisis talks with our head of fundraising; do we press the button on a significant investment in Russia for our mobile phone insurance business; sign-off on new website concepts and logo designs for our 25th anniversary; plan my week in the US – this is a big one with stops in New York, Miami, Dallas, Houston, LA; back to the office for my weekly meeting with our CTO; and finally dash out to the car just after 7pm to get to a dinner with either friends, a school function, a visiting executive or potential investors…150 emails have come in during the meeting mania.

I write this not to impress you but to describe what I am sure is a typical day for a "C" level executive these days. We run very hard and I work 60-70 hours per week. I will have completed 70 flights in the year when I return to London to start 2013. Work-life balance – does it exist? Can it exist? The reality is that if you are over 40 years old and successful in business, the chances are you work very hard and play very hard. It seems to be the reality of our modern business society. So what is work-life balance for this group of people?

I am going to defy the traditional view here and say for the record – sorry gentleman, you cannot and will not ever have work-life balance if you are a driven and successful man at the top of his game. I don't believe it is possible. There are some super successful guys who have made it big and have achieved the ultimate balance, but they are rare and in a small minority – I congratulate you and you inspire me.

However, for 99.9% of us, the reality is we are going to continue to work incredibly hard to maintain our careers and our lifestyles. We are going to be stressed, we are going to compromise our health, we are going to take our partners for granted, we are going to neglect our kids, we are going to be exhausted by the time the weekend comes around, we are going to keep obsessing with our smart phones and we will likely drop at some point – mentally, physically or both.

I genuinely believe there is a better way, and am not going to give you a spiel about traditional work-life balance, meditation, cut down the hours, don't do as much next year, give up alcohol, go to the gym, get those golf lessons, take the kids to school once a week, etc. In my world, I am a CEO of a successful business and as I have mentioned I work long hours (by choice). I love what I do and keep pushing the envelope. I am also an age-nostic man and have been inspired by Michael Hogg, his journey and his vision for a better way to age and enjoy the second half of our lives. Not every one who reads this book will have lived the extremes Michael has, but I absolutely recommend you devour the content because we can all identify with it and learn so much from his journey and his wisdom on how to age better.

The Lessons

What I am going to give you here is a series of lessons learned over the past 20 years of my career that I believe will really help a lot of men who find themselves in a situation where they are still going for it. First, I am going to give you a formula:
Reality = no such thing as work-life balance for a successful driven man
Solution = be smarter with your time, and you will be happier and healthier

Other lessons learned:

1. *Be ruthless with your time.*
2. *Executive assistants are gold – treat them well.*
3. *Get your personal and professional goals in sync.*
4. *Find out how to sleep well.*
5. *Quantity versus quality with loved ones.*
6. *If you are going to be there – be there.*
   No matter how trivial – look interested, be interested.
   They just want some of you.
7. *You are no longer Superman nor are you Mr. Gray.*
8. *Clear the personal cache – me time.*
9. *Stay connected – it causes more stress if you don't.*
10. *What you put in your mouth catches up with you.*
11. *Take the time to:*
    Take yourself shopping;
    Have a facial;
    Buy face creams and that sort of stuff, even if you don't use it – it feels good.
12. *Dare to be different – the element of surprise.*
13. *Whatever you do – fly and travel smarter.*
    Minimum business class where possible, especially long haul.
    Don't walk straight into a meeting.
    Get a good night's sleep.
14. *Know where you stand – get yourself properly tested top to toe.*

The 21st-Century Workplace

Some theorists suggest that this blurred boundary of work and life is a result of technology alone, but I have always felt it's caused by a number of inter-connected factors. Newspapers, social media and even our schooling help promote the need to be as good as or better than the next person. Whatever the cause, work has entered our whole lives. It is clear that problems caused by stress have become a major concern to both employers and employees. Symptoms of stress are manifested, both physiologically and psychologically, and should never be swept under the carpet. Persistent high levels of stress can result in all sorts of personal problems such as a weaker immune system, headaches, stiff muscles and/ or our sexual health. It can also result in growing feelings of insecurity, exhaustion and difficulty concentrating. Stress may also lead to a greater likelihood of developing dependent and addictive behaviour as we get older with the likes of smoking, overeating and other disorders.

Some employers believe that workers should reduce their own stress levels by making a better effort to care for their own health and simplify their lives. I have certainly seen cases where the chief cause of stress has been a company and the behaviour of its management. More men are realizing that work is not the only source of fulfillment in their life, which can be a major help in fighting against stress. More of us are looking for greater flexibility just as much as women. However, with an ever-changing society, flexibility is becoming much more apparent and not always easy to organize.

The state of our mental health is a balancing act that may be affected by a number of inter-related factors. I believe the four key ones are as follows:

1. *Genes* – some of us are born with less favourable genes when it comes to mental health.

2. *Major trauma* – when we have experienced a major event such as a death in the family or loss of a job.

3. *Inward pressure* – the pressure we put on ourselves to achieve goals and reach targets, which are often unattainable.

4. *Stress* – others putting us under pressure to achieve or do things. This may inadvertently be our partner, family members or friends.

Many people are exposed to job stress, because the "hard worker" seems to enjoy, among other things, very high social recognition in many workplaces. It's a feeling that because someone works really long hours, they must be important and vital to the cause. Most studies I have read place a strong link between pressure in the workplace and increased amounts of stress in society. What we strive to achieve in the workplace seems to be increasingly important in the balance of our mental well-being.

As our lives have become busier, finding the right work-life balance for us as individuals has also become tougher. It is a moving target for a start, although usually there are underlying trends in our behaviour and outlook, which cannot be ignored. Technology has made our lives so much easier, faster and more personal. We can speak to people any time of the night or day, tell a whole group what we are up to at any minute and find out facts at the click of a button. We seemingly can't live without our smart phones, tablets, e-readers, portable computers and the rest.

The downside has yet to be fully explored or understood, as we also now struggle to switch off and be out of reach when work wants something. It turns us into completely reactive animals. We no longer spend the same amount of time thinking and analyzing whether things are actually good for us, as we are too busy reacting to the constant stream of incoming noise. A good friend of mine was having problems seeing the wood from the company trees: his relationship was going through a bad patch and he could not seem to prioritize properly. I had a drink with him after work one evening and asked him to try something. I said he should see the next weekend as the time to think and re-set his priorities to his own agenda. I'm not sure if he managed to do this the whole weekend, but I told him to switch off his iPhone and not look at any emails. I tried to get him to not look at the television but Rome wasn't built in a day. He did get a blank pad of paper and started to list the things that made up his life. When he had the list, I asked him to prioritize what would be really important to him over the next 10 years. Not all of his troubles were sorted out by Sunday evening, but I feel he made great strides and turned a corner. We laugh about it now but we both know it helped a lot.

Anyone who has worked with me knows I find getting the balance right in my life one of the toughest things. I get enthusiastic about a project and working with people and other things get left behind. I am certainly not holding myself up as a shining light in this space at all. I did meet a business author and small-time entrepreneur recently who started his own business in his late 30s just so he could have greater control over his own work-life relationship. He had several opportunities to grow the small central London operation but declined each time. His view was that he enjoyed the more personal and intimate running of his small business and he felt he was driving it, not someone else. Making it larger would mean him spending more time doing the things he didn't want to do. In terms of avoiding a mid-life crisis, there is a lot to be said for putting work-life balance high up on your career and life agenda.

Ten tips for coping with a mid-life crisis:

1. The worse shape you are in, the harder it will be.
2. You will go through a crisis – all of us eventually do.
3. Do not lose the child in you.
4. Get some younger friends.
5. Don't panic.
6. Reassess your life goals.
7. Follow this book and choose the level you want to get to.
8. The rules are: there are no rules!
9. The next 10 years will see a transformation in ageing.
10. Refuse to accept the norm.

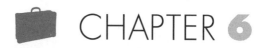

CHAPTER **6**

KICKING THE BLACK DOG OF LIFE

Understanding depression and how to cope with it

It is no longer as hard to talk about depression because it seems to be such an everyday topic in today's media and society. It doesn't take long for someone well known to come out and admit to their own depressive illness and how it has so dramatically affected their life. The absolute darkness it brings upon them is something I understand and will very reluctantly outline here, hoping it will show you how it can be beaten.

Later in this chapter, I will tell you exactly what I do to protect myself when I see the black dog of depression approaching and what I do day-to-day to make sure it passes by more times than it stops. But first, how did it start? Looking back now, it is hard to understand the actual events and reasons that took me into the black hole. It started when I literally had a functioning breakdown. I didn't have a full, take-him-away meltdown, but I am sure now it was the next best thing. In the space of a few months, my life changed in every way possible.

It was Christmas 2008, and my wife and I had just moved into our new house and planned a big house-warming party to celebrate. I had been travelling (or running away) far too much as usual, and my drinking had reached dangerous levels with huge intermittent binges while I was in London. I had been spending time on my own which was never productive mentally. I returned to Sydney as we were moving into the new house and was, as usual, very jet-lagged. As the guests filled the house, I proceeded to get very drunk very quickly, something that happened a lot when I was exhausted. I enjoyed the party immensely – who wouldn't with all that self-medication?

I remember sitting on our new balcony in the morning, the sun up, drinking a beer. My wife got up, came out to see me sitting there and said nothing except, "Do you want some coffee?" I came inside and said to her, "I think I am having some sort of breakdown". Looking back, it was the last time she ever put her arms around me. She had had enough and it was not long after that day I would pack my suitcase and walk up the driveway of my new home, never to return.

I was totally lost by now but didn't realize it then, and the next six months were going to be a descent into what could only be described as complete darkness. I moved into a flat that I had owned at the time, a small studio on Bondi beach with a beautiful view of the surf, which was at least a start. Not that I noticed the surf much; I saw very little of beauty in those twilight days. I was starting to sink each day into a fog. I was having trouble getting out of bed but tried to get myself moving in any direction at all. I was fast losing hope that I was ever going to feel normal again, and managed to stumble through without too many people seeing the severe problems I was having. Looking back, this was a true performance worthy of an academy award.

One big step forward was getting a girlfriend. I was in the first serious relationship since the breakdown of my marriage, having met a wonderful girl on a blind date set up by a close friend. She was already noticing my binge drinking and the writing was on the wall. The relationship would only last six months due to my emotional highs and lows, and this proved to be the trigger for me to step into the deepest hole. One day I was driving and received a call from my father's cleaner who sounded very distressed. She said she had found my father lying on the floor of his apartment and thought he was dead. She had managed to get him conscious but he looked in a bad way. I told her I would be straight over and to call the paramedics. I arrived a short time later to see the paramedics over him trying to get him to talk while giving him oxygen. The apartment was like something out of the movies, with dozens of empty wine bottles stacked up everywhere. Later I was to find every cupboard totally full of empty wine bottles and nothing else. I guess he had been hiding them rather than putting them out with the garbage.

His body was hugely bloated and it was hard to recognize the big personality that had brought me up. I was only to find out later when he was in hospital that he had been in that position for days. He had taken an overdose of anti-depressants and sleeping pills that should have killed anyone. I feared for my own future and only later did my counsellor explain to me that he had given me a gift by showing me a snapshot of my own future. It was very hard for me to see a previously strong man end up in such a hopeless situation.

I am pleased to say that after a lot more pain and heartache, he is still alive and finally reasonably happy, living in an old people's home. He has had his 80th birthday and has found the right medication to allow him to function reasonably normally. I tried my best to understand what he must have gone through to get into that state but was very angry at him (this had happened before). This period distracted me somewhat from my own problems, but it was not long before I fell back into the black hole.

I needed a change of scenery to help me feel more positive, so decided to move into a bigger place, a terraced house in the suburb of Paddington in Sydney. They are traditionally rather dark homes and I guess I chose a place that reflected my own mood. Looking back, that probably wasn't the smartest decision I ever made. I was not functioning at work at all and decided to resign from my job running this huge company. I just couldn't get on another plane and had lost my motivation to continue. I called Chris and told him. He was disappointed but understanding.

I had now cut off another artery of stability. Work had helped me hugely over the years with self-esteem and also a way to deflect some of my worst inner feelings. My possible escape routes from myself had also diminished as I didn't have to travel to London anymore. This just left me with my own thoughts of despair, which were only building in intensity on a daily basis. I now felt truly alone, which is what I seemed to desire. Here I was with my beloved canine, having left my home, family and career as well as trying to understand my father's demise. My mother had died a few years before from lung cancer and heavy drinking, which was a terrible way to go. I started not going out of the house for days, which turned into weeks, and I was getting seriously depressed. My dear friend, Michael Zacharia, suggested that I might try medication, but I was absolutely terrified of prescription drugs after what had happened to my father. I refused any suggestions point blank.

Eventually, I did take some valium at times when the panic got so bad, but quickly worked out that it doesn't go too well with a bottle of red wine. One night I woke up on the couch totally disorientated to find Gypsie (my dog) curled up on my shoulder staring at me. She was to be a good friend over the coming months and somehow never left my side among all the madness. I am sure she knew what was happening.

The coming months were simply a battle to stay in control and get through each day. It an amazing hour-by-hour existence when you are in a very depressive state and days take forever to pass. For a few weeks I was self-medicating each night with alcohol as my world became darker and darker. Eventually I came to realize I was waking up feeling even worse than before, and this got me to stop drinking completely. At times, alcohol had been a useful sedative, and in the immediate aftermath without it I entered the most terrifying period of my life. I started not sleeping and staying up all night for days, pacing around the house (with Gypsie always following me). I started telling myself to hang on as I really thought I was going mad. Up to that point in my life, I had always slept well and it was a horrible and unnerving feeling to see the sun come up, realizing that you had not slept at all.

I don't know exactly how many weeks this went on for but it seemed like months. Each evening came after a long empty day, and I was getting completely paranoid about the night time arriving because I knew it would contain hours of me talking to myself. I was too depressed to call anyone and felt ashamed. Even when my kids would call me, I would try somehow to sound normal, but I was avoiding them as well. They were going through their own issues with the marriage break-up and I just didn't want to worry them.

After many weeks of this, my body and mind were completely exhausted and I wasn't even dressing or shaving anymore. I felt like Howard Hughes in the movie *The Aviator*, sitting in a room for days (at least he had heaps of money) and not coming out. I honestly thought I was going mad, but somehow I could just about manage to put on a façade of normality when I saw my friends and kids. That is one of the remarkable things about depressed people. They look normal, with no outward scars, marks or burns, because all the damage is inside and can be smoothed over for short periods of time.

I did manage to see a counsellor and he could tell that I was having a meltdown, having done a lot of crying on his couch and confused thinking. One day I got dressed in my suit and went into Sydney without any plan at all. I ended up sitting on a bench in Hyde Park for most of the day, unable to move at all. I knew I was really in trouble and totally froze as I did not know what to do. I was finally at the end. I thought of going to hospital but could not work out what I would say, and I didn't want to let anyone down, especially my kids.

I was just about managing to do some work part-time and needed to keep a little money coming in, so the fewer people that knew, the better.

It was getting towards the end of the day, but I couldn't leave that bench. I didn't know which direction to go. I was a bit over-dressed for an overnight stay in the park, so I called my counsellor. He told me he thought I had indeed reached the end and to book myself into hospital. I flatly refused (like father, like son) but it did get me off that bench. My counsellor ran a great programme called the Hoffman Process, which focuses on family relationships and how they help to shape our lives. He suggested I join the next programme starting in Byron Bay as he thought it might help. I booked and paid, and got a friend, Christian (who had been looking after me through the really bad days), to drive me to the airport. I got on the plane and off I went. This trip was to change my life and probably save it.

The Recovery

The course and its content were fascinating and gave me an insight into my own childhood and early influences. A combination of the people around and the daily distractions, together with good healthy food and plenty of self-examination, allowed me to get my thinking back on track. I had been surfing the Net late at night when I was not sleeping, learning as much as I could about depression. I was determined to get through without having to resort to anti-depressants. I was amazed to find how big the subject had become and how much information was available.

I quickly identified that there were many supplements one could take to alleviate and lift the low mood that comes along with depression. I learned about 5http L tryptophan, fish oil, pre-gaba, pre-dopa and the wonder lifter, magnesium. I also found out how certain foods can cause us to slip into a depressive state and there are many that can get us out. Other helpful supplements which were widely used in many parts of the world increase the levels of serotonin and dopamine dramatically which in return helps us to lift ourselves out of depression. I established that alcohol and most self-medication, while providing quick relief, was the worst thing we could do when we are feeling low, as after a short high, it will only make us feel even lower.

When I returned to Sydney after the week-long course, I was feeling a lot better. But as soon as I got back to the emptiness of my house, the feelings of despair immediately returned. I fell into a panic that the whole cycle was going to repeat itself, with even more serious results. However, I managed to convince myself I could make it through another bout, which proved to be the turning point in my life. I chose not to go back but to move forward and fight each day. I became more excited as I felt better and better. I started eating foods that would lift me and undertook an exercise regime every day. I found this especially helpful as a routine to start the morning, when depression tends to be at its worst.

I had learned transcendental meditation over 20 years ago but had stopped using it. I started practising again for the required 20 minutes and it had a huge effect on me. What amazed me most was how quickly I came out of the fog, and after only a couple of weeks I was feeling much improved. I slowly re-entered the world of normal people, and the silver lining was being able to appreciate so many of the smaller things. I was just so happy to feel positive again, and to this day I have never been back to that totally dark place. That is not to say I don't get hit with depressive episodes on occasions, because I do. However, what I have learned from this whole experience is that you must have an effective way to deal with, and shorten, the bad times. On most occasions now I can rid myself of the black dog very quickly.

This was my own story of the black dog. I am now going to let an expert in psychology have his say and provide us with a deeper insight into the subject.

The Psychology of Depression
By Tim Watson-Munro

Depression is becoming more recognized and socially acceptable as an illness. Notwithstanding this, many in the community still feel stigmatized by the diagnosis, and from my clinical experience this appears to be particularly relevant to men in their mid-life cycle. Depression is not just about feeling sad, but rather reflects a major chemical imbalance in the brain referable to depletions of vital neurotransmitters responsible for the regulation of mood. These primarily include dopamine and serotonin, and many of the drug treatments of choice assist the brain in retaining these neurochemicals to maintain a buoyant mood. Pharmacologically, they are described as Selective Serotonin Reuptake Inhibitors (SSRIs). The first of these to hit the market was Prozac, which was greeted with much enthusiasm and acclaim in 1987. Since then, SSRIs have been further refined and for some have proven to be of considerable benefit in terms of offsetting the persistent feelings of despair, thoughts of suicide, low levels of energy and drive and sexual dysfunction, which are often prime indices of a major depressive illness.

There is a significant difference between day-to-day sadness arising from stressful life events, such as the loss of a loved one or job, and major depression, which becomes an all-pervasive illness affecting more than just mood. In general, it affects all aspects of the sufferer's life, including energy levels, perception of reality, capacity to plan, control impulses and maintaining sound judgment.

In over 34 years of clinical practice and academic life, I have encountered many thousands of examples of depressive illness and its impact upon the patient, with sufferers often being transformed into individuals who are plagued with chronic feelings of self-doubt, worthlessness, irritability, avoidant behaviour, substantial sleep disturbance and a tendency to act in many and varied bizarre ways.

My own depressive illness erupted out of the blue, or so it seemed. In retrospect I came to realize that it had been percolating for many years as a consequence of working inordinately long hours and the very nature of my employment, which has involved assessing psychopathic offenders who have committed horrendous crimes. During the course of my career, I have been involved in excess of 200 murder trials as well as the so-called "Hoddle Street Massacre" in Melbourne which, at the time, was the largest mass murder in Australian criminal history. This case represented a double-edged sword and reflected a watershed in my career. On the one hand, it placed me in a situation of national prominence, which in turn established my credentials in the field; but on the other, at a more subtle level due to the nature of the material I was required to assess and digest, it dramatically transformed my view of the world and its inhabitants.

As a consequence of spending most of my working hours dealing with the "dark side" of human nature, my previously spontaneous, creative and happy disposition was gradually eroded to a point where I was plagued with feelings of cynicism, self-doubt and an underlying sense of resentment. As time progressed, my energy levels began to dissipate, as did my motivation for the work. I had previously been highly enthusiastic about my career and certainly had reveled in the publicity, which I had received attendant to the many high-profile cases I had been involved in throughout Australia. To those who knew me, I wore a public façade of self-confidence, success and wealth. In my quieter hours, however, I genuinely believed that my success was nothing more than a "con" and that I lacked any real ability in terms of my capacity as a forensic psychologist. This contributed to feelings of guilt, despair and ever-dwindling self-confidence. The seeds of my depressive illness were fully harvested when, in short succession, my first wife, Susan, was diagnosed with terminal bowel cancer in approximately 1998. Although we had been divorced for a number of years, we had enjoyed a loving and amicable relationship as reflected in the fact that we shared custody of our children and I continued to support her at a level of financial significance. The news of her illness and its inevitable consequence shattered what was left of my attempts to maintain a reasonably buoyant mood. The situation was compounded by the fact that we had two young children who were approaching adolescence. Although I was well supported by my current partner, Carla Lechner, this in itself was insufficient for me to overcome my difficulties.

As is so often the case with middle-aged men and particularly those who are successful, I refused to seek treatment in the first instance and to disclose the extent of my despair. By this stage, a prior pattern of occasionally using cocaine dramatically escalated as a means of self-medication, with this in turn affecting my capacity to make rational decisions on occasion as well as exacerbating my depression. I felt great shame concerning my addiction but due to my public profile, felt hopeless in terms of seeking professional assistance and disclosing the extent of my problems, as I feared it would become public knowledge. For a time, suicide seemed the only rational choice for me although I was held back by my love for my children and partner. In addition to my profession, I had previously enjoyed playing classical guitar and piano, which I had studied from an early age, and reading and listening to music. But now I found myself *often sleeping for days at a time, unable to get out of bed and cancelling appointments. Fortunately I had employed a competent psychologist to assist me and in this context my tracks were covered for a time.*

In retrospect, my situation was not unique and certainly since resuming my practice some years ago, I frequently encounter middle-aged men experiencing similar problems. This, no doubt, is a result of a combination of events including faulty neurochemistry, life stressors and a feeling in these men that their best years are behind them.

Middle age represents a major turning point and potential time of crisis for many men. This has been described somewhat dismissively as a "mid-life crisis", but in my own view it represents a far more serious condition for many of us. It comes at a time when sexual potency and sense of attractiveness decreases, a sense of ageing increases and our health begins to decline in subtle ways. This is reflected in weight gain, reduced energy and drive, a sense of boredom in work and, often with men who suffer depression, significant marital tension. It is often unrecognized and consequently undiagnosed and untreated. It is against this backdrop that potentially more serious and life-threatening behaviours develop.

As a consequence, some men may drift into patterns of alcohol or substance misuse as a means of self-medication. The paradox relates to alcohol being a central nervous system depressant, which in turn aggravates the individual's underlying depressive illness beyond brief periods of respite when they are intoxicated and dissociated from their problems. Other individuals, including myself at that time, resort to drug abuse. In my case, my drug of choice was cocaine because it energized me and provided a feeling of infallibility (albeit a false one), which acted as a guard against my underlying feelings of inadequacy referable to my cognition being affected because of my depression.

It is on this basis that individuals quickly acquire an addiction to alcohol or drugs, because in the absence of these substances, troubling thoughts and biochemical depression resumes. In terms of cocaine and these days, crystal methylamphetamine ("ice"), which is frequently used among middle-class professionals, the depletion of dopamine and serotonin which is released in turbo-charged quantities leads to a severe depletion of mood regulators for days at a time. These fuel depression, leading to further use. As has so often been said, "one line is too many and a thousand is never enough". Stimulant drugs also lead to sleep disturbance, which in turn can cause significant impairment of an individual's capacity to negotiate their lives. Irritability with a low threshold for frustration and general fractiousness is very common. Alcohol and drug abusers spend their lives dealing with high levels of anxiety when not euphoric, and with the passage of time develop severe paranoia and, on occasion, even psychotic breaks including delusions as well as auditory and visual hallucinations. There is now significant scientific evidence to suggest that with protracted stimulant drug abuse, subtle organic changes occur in the prefrontal cortex of the brain, a structure that is responsible for higher cognitive executive functioning. The sufferer consequently drifts into a pattern of an increasingly diminished capacity to cope with their lives, thus fuelling their despair and depression and anxiety.

This affliction should be recognized as a genuine psychiatric disorder in the Western world, for these drugs are still abused, as reflected in statistics coming out of Europe, the United States and Australia. I am seeing a significant number of men holding highly responsible and well-paid positions in public and private companies who concede that they have closet addictions to cocaine and "ice" which they use to stay awake and maintain heavy workloads. As a consequence of the information technology revolution, our brains are constantly bombarded with data 24 hours a day, seven days a week. Some experts have recently suggested that addiction to technology, including the Internet and other communication devices and games, should be recognized as a major psychiatric disorder. At a more proximal level, it leads to there never being any quiet time for men to enjoy domestic life with their families. Being frequently harassed on the weekends via emails and mobile telephone calls leaves no free time for quiet contemplation and reflection. There is evidence to suggest that our brains are unable to cope with the rapid changes in technology that have led to the information revolution. This in turn feeds into the despair and anxiety that I have described referable to the vicious treadmill of work stress, substance abuse, depletion of neurochemicals and mental illness compounded by alcohol and substance misuse. Inevitably, the changes in cognition and behaviour, which result in the confluence of these factors, lead to marital discord and disharmony at work. On occasions this can lead a person to fall foul of the law, destroy their marriage and indeed lose their career. There is often a strong interface between depression, anxiety and low self-esteem. I have encountered many individuals over the years who, despite an outward persona of very successful professional and family lives, have suffered longstanding feelings of inadequacy which can be traced back to their formative childhood years. It can arise from under-bonding with their parents, absent father and mother figures, marital breakdown, demographic dislocation impacting upon schooling, and in some instances physical, psychological and sexual abuse at the hands of step-parents. Without wishing to appear arrogant, with some 34 years' experience in the field, I have reached a point where I can generally tell if a person has come from a broken home when they walk into my consulting room. I think there is little argument that an intact family unit ultimately, if the partners can work through their difficulties, is in the best interests of children and their healthy psychological development. In the absence of this, they develop feelings of deep insecurity, resentment, hostility and low self-esteem, which in turn can be aggravated if they are frequently moved from school to school. Arising from this, they are deprived of the opportunity to establish meaningful peer group relationships.

The treatment for mood disorders and depression are numerous and varied. While I know and respect that Michael Hogg has not chosen this, generally the first line of attack relates to anti-depressant medication. Although in individuals with severe depression improvements can be gained through these types of drugs, it is the case for many that it takes some time to find the right type of anti-depressant for the individual. Anti-depressants also take some time to take effect in terms of therapeutic efficacy. More often than not there are side effects attached to these medications, which include a substantial reduction in libido, difficulties with ejaculation, other sexual dysfunction, and a sense of dissociation from one's environment. Some individuals complain of weight gain, headaches and nausea and as a consequence may become non-compliant with their treatment. This, in turn, leads to a recrudescence of their despair and a belief that they are beyond help, contributing to an ultimate feeling of hopelessness. When a man loses hope and dignity, he has little to live for, and as a result may then become actively suicidal. This catch-22 referable to conventional psychotropic medication for depression and anxiety requires *further research and refinement. In the interim, however, there are alternative therapies that can assist a male to regain his sense of self, improve his self-esteem, his sexual functioning and his capacity to relate to others. Believe it or not, based on my own experience, eventually individuals can once again enjoy their careers.*

In closing, one of the major obstacles that I found needed to be overcome related to the general tendency of men to shut down their emotions, particularly when they are troubled. As a gender, we need to learn to communicate more with those around us who are in a strong position to provide immense emotional support, if only we can let them in. In the alternative, the ongoing process of repressing one's feelings is highly corrosive and generally leads to acting out in strange and elusive ways, such as buying a Harley-Davidson motorcycle, an MGB or taking up paragliding in one's 50s. It is important that we learn to forgive ourselves for mistakes and forgive others, in order to avoid continuously beating ourselves up for past mistakes. Eventually you will reach a position of feeling far more comfortable in your own skin, which then better equips you to deal with life as it stands today and in the future, rather than dwelling in a moribund state reflecting upon the past.

How to Tackle Depression

To begin with, I would advise having a good look back at your family history to see if there are any patterns of depression or anything similar. This may not necessarily mean you will suffer from it, but there is a lot of evidence to suggest that many forms of depression could well be hereditary. Whether there is a physiological and/or environmental link, no one is certain, and I don't think the experts have come up with any definitive answer to date. So little worthwhile research exists, which in turn has held back treatment for many years.

If depression is going to appear in your life, it is more likely to happen in your mid-life years. This is a time when many men are not in the best physical shape to combat problems and many factors such as diet, alcohol, career, family changes, etc. can contribute to an increased likelihood of depression. After we reach 40 years of age, things start to look more challenging generally.

As we face the challenges of ageing, the mind can easily get filled with doubt and apprehension about the future. This phase of life and what it can bring represents a time of great uncertainty for most men.

We should, however, recognize the symptoms of real depression, as opposed to simple feelings of sadness or lack of enthusiasm for life. Too many people run off to their doctor thinking they are suffering from depression, when they may in fact be going through a particularly rough period in their life. There is a very big difference between the two and I, for one, can relate to that happening on more than one occasion.

Symptoms of depression vary with each individual and can also change over time, but here is a general guide:

1. Persistent sad, anxious or "empty" moods.
2. Feelings of hopelessness or pessimism.
3. Feelings of guilt, worthlessness or lack of purpose.
4. Loss of interest or pleasure in hobbies and activities that were once enjoyed, including sex.
5. Decreased energy, fatigue or a feeling of "slowing down".
6. Difficulty concentrating, remembering or making decisions.
7. Insomnia, early-morning awakening or oversleeping.
8. Appetite and/or weight loss or over-eating and weight gain.
9. Thoughts of death or actual suicide attempts.
10. Restlessness or irritability.

So what can we do to arrest this situation? First, don't get too carried away with the whole depression thing. If we believe what is written in the press, it would appear that the whole Western world is plunging into a depressive state. The statistics on the number of people taking anti-depressants are truly astounding, and one would actually think that the above is true. I believe that thinking you are clinically depressed can actually make you depressed. After all, feeling depressed is quite a depressing feeling and it can all become a self-fulfilling prophecy if you are not careful.

It is only recently that world leaders have been exposed as drug takers of some kind. The most notable were President John F. Kennedy, Adolf Hitler and Winston Churchill who were all addicted to amphetamines during their

tenure at the top, and who all suffered from depression. I have never been on anti-depressant drugs, nor will I ever go on them. My view is that no matter how bad I feel, I will never be able to take the step of going on medication that may well lift me out of depression in the short term, but is likely to lead to long-term reliance. Besides, two of the biggest side effects of most anti-depressants are weight gain and loss of sexual drive, and the chance of those two side effects occurring is enough for me to stay away. Both have a considerable impact on our levels of self-esteem and confidence.

If you think you are depressed or becoming depressed and have been for some time, I would recommend the following before taking any further action:

1. Don't panic.
2. Don't convince yourself you are depressed.
3. Analyze what has happened in your life to make you feel this way (one-off incident or a range of things).
4. Stay away from all self-medication as much as possible, especially alcohol.
5. No matter how bad you feel, especially in the morning, do some exercise.
6. Do not stay in bed after normal sleeping hours.
7. Only eat foods that lift depression and avoid foods that manifest the depressive feelings.
8. Manage it and accept it.
9. Don't go off medication immediately without medical supervision just because you are feeling better for a period (especially prescribed medication).
10. Hopefully you will use medication as a last resort – there are better ways.

One of my favourite sayings, which I always refer to during bad times, is "And this too will pass". It always does when we look back on life, as most crises we deal with are relatively temporary.

The bottom line is simple: most men will experience at least one period in their life (likely to be when they are over 40) where they feel overwhelmed and are convinced that they are depressed. The whole moral of this chapter is give everything mentioned in this book a try before you race off to the doctor or the nearest bridge. If nothing works, then of course go and see your doctor, who will happily prescribe you some medication to make you feel better and make the world look brighter. The trick then will be to get off that medication once you are feeling better, although this can be a difficult challenge even for the strongest among us.

Ten tips for coping with depression:

1. It's completely normal to feel depressed at times.
2. But it's not normal to be depressed at all times.
3. Eat foods that combat depression.
4. Don't eat foods that make depression worse.
5. Watch what you drink and how much.
6. Take supplements that stimulate serotonin and dopamine.
7. Treat anti-depressants as a last resort.
8. Don't feel ashamed when the "black dog" hits – talk to someone!
9. Exercise even when you don't feel like it.
10. Seek medical help if you have tried all of the above without success.

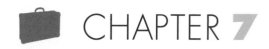

CHAPTER 7

ADDICTIVE BEHAVIOUR

More than just a few lines

If you can honestly say you have no addiction problems, or any form of addictive behaviour, then you can probably skip this chapter. However, if you are like the majority of men in their 40s and beyond, you may want to read on and see if there are any familiar signs. Statistics show that the problem of addiction is significant in this age group, and the point of this chapter is not to get you to hit the panic button and send you rushing off to rehab, but increase awareness of how careful you need to be.

As a teenager in the 1970s, I was like many who simply drank a lot, which seemed to be accepted, if not expected. There was no education on alcohol abuse whatsoever, and I came from a fairly affluent home where there was always alcohol around. It was a time of freedom, drinking was cool and a big part of life, even at home. In my case, much of my father's business activities in those days were conducted at home through cocktail receptions, dinner parties and endless socializing.

When I was 10 to 15 years old, life was full of exciting and interesting things. My parents would always make sure we came in to say hello to all the guests and everyone was always so happy and vibrant. The drinks would always be flowing and I learned at an early age that people simply had fun when they drank. I would go to bed and listen to the din of noise coming from the entertainment and the excitement would slowly increase. The fabulous tones of Barry White, who was hugely popular in those days, would get louder as the night went on and I used to lie awake listening to the glasses clinking. I so wanted to be part of it.

I would get up in the morning and go into the lounge to view the debris. What fun they must have had, I thought, to cause such a mess. At times, I could hear my parents arguing about something or other, which was unusual because they never argued during the day. At that time I didn't understand that it was my mother's drinking that was causing the arguments. I couldn't wait to be part of this lifestyle, and before long I was getting up after a typical

Saturday night party to sample some of the leftovers. Back then, everyone drank gin and tonic.

Other occasions perpetuated this feeling in me. Christmas Day was always an exciting trip back to New Zealand to see the family, which was quite large. I still recall those wonderful gatherings and everyone drank enormous amounts of alcohol. My mum and dad drank every night, although my mum always more. It was in my teens that I started noticing drinking seemed to change her personality as she became much more aggressive and confrontational. She would talk about basically nothing and slur her words, but it didn't quite register to someone so young that this was abnormal. I was getting unwittingly conditioned without knowing it.

As I became an older teenager, my mother used to have what she called Friday night drinks with her girlfriends, which meant a drinks party at some friend's house where I would be invited already. This usually started at 5pm and always ended at about 7.30pm when dad called to see where she was. Mum would then be put into her VW Beetle and would drive slowly home. Mum would chain smoke in the car, happy as a lark, and I started to realize she was completely drunk. How we got home safely most Fridays was a miracle looking back now. But again, I loved the social gathering, and there were always children of our own age around and no one bothered us. All the mothers were having too good a time, with gin flowing and cigarettes being lit continuously.

The men were all doing the same, often during the day as the long business lunch scene continued to prosper. I always remember dad could never stay awake when he came home. He used to sit down in his chair and fall asleep. I never saw him as being drunk and thought it was just because he had worked hard all day. As my final years of school came to an end, every weekend was one long party. I was at one of Sydney's best private schools and all the homes we visited were large with a pool. Parents loved to open their homes to us kids as it was a great excuse for them to party as well. Everyone got drunk and there were always incidents, mainly with people falling into pools. When we could drive, we all used to drive home drunk as there was no one to pull us over in those days.

My early years of work and travel were exciting and the parties were endless. I never noticed if I drank more than anyone else; after all, everyone drank so much, it was impossible to tell. We were young and fit and hangovers were just cured by heading to the beach to surf. We were too young to feel whether we were becoming addicted and our bodies too strong to show the effects. How different it is later in life. This went on for many years, as work relationships and life rolled into one and it wasn't until much later that the warning bells began to ring.

When I returned from my crazy adventures in the Philippines, I went to stay with my mother for a while. Over the years I noticed her drinking getting worse, and her changing, but she always looked amazing. She loved being around young people and would often come to the many parties we had in our late 20s. Everyone loved her, but incidents started occurring that caused my brother and I a lot of embarrassment. She just wouldn't ever leave a party. Mum was the most incredible person most of the time but when she had too much to drink, which was most nights while I stayed with her, a dark side came out.

I am constantly amazed at how much alcohol many of us actually consume, and it is so rare to meet anyone that doesn't drink alcohol. It is also a common thread among highly successful people, creative types and entrepreneurs that drinking to excess is more the norm than the exception. I am never sure whether addiction is a genetic disposition or an environmental consequence from our early learning. I am sure for most people it is a bit of both, but take a good look at your own patterns and background. I am sure that if you have a family history of heavy drinkers or worse, it is well worth being aware of your own possible tendencies.

There is no doubt in my mind that the years after 40 are a watershed for any addiction development or movement into a chronic situation. This is simply the worst time to find out you may have a serious problem as your body and mind will find it so much harder to recover. The sudden slide into a position where there is no way back can be very fast indeed. I know all too well the direct relationship between depression and alcohol abuse. Do we drink because we get depressed or get depressed because we drink? The same can be said for drug taking, eating disorders and others. Self-medicating because of depression, while offering brief relief, is undoubtedly the worst thing we can possibly do. This is because depression in the longer term only gets worse as the result of alcohol because it is a depressant, even though many people think it is the opposite.

We heard earlier from psychologist Tim Watson-Munro about his experience of depression. Here he continues his story by focusing on the addictive behaviour side, and ultimately his remarkable fall from grace and rise again.

To Cocaine and Back

By Tim Watson-Munro

One day, I was attending a birthday party for one of Australia's leading Queen's Counsels, Philip Dunn QC, when word filtered through the backyard of his home regarding a mutual colleague. This person, Andrew Roderick Fraser, who was also a criminal lawyer, had been arrested by the Victorian and Australian Federal Police in relation to a conspiracy to import 6 kilograms of high-quality cocaine into the country. Fraser, at that stage, was a close mate of most of us in the medico-legal fraternity and, indeed, had briefed me in my capacity as a forensic psychologist on many occasions. To this end, we had shared many years plying our respective fields of expertise to various cases including the America's Cup hero, Alan Bond, the Melbourne Construction giant, Bruno Grollo, and the disgraced former Chairman of Coles-Myer, Brian Quinn.

All of the hubris associated with success vapourized in that instant with the news of Fraser's arrest. As with many areas of commerce, gossip is the life-blood of the criminal justice system and it was not long before the news had spread like wild-fire throughout the Victorian legal fraternity. It singularly and collectively feasted on the professional carcass of Fraser or as he is now commonly described, "ARF the dog", Andrew Roderick Fraser.

Arising from this devastating development, particularly in the context of having no knowledge of his involvement with importing this insidious drug, I realized I was in deep trouble. During the course of our relationship, both ARF and I had become involved in using cocaine. I consequently realized at that moment that my days as a practising forensic psychologist could be numbered.

Although at no stage had there been any suggestion that I was implicated or had knowledge of the cocaine importation, the Victorian Police Force nonetheless was now aware of my habit and, in particular, that I had purchased the drug from Fraser. Adding to my panic, I knew it was just a question of time before the press became involved, and as a consequence my wife, children, close friends and those who had held me in such high regard for many years would no doubt be shattered by the revelation of my dual life.

I first started practising in Melbourne in 1981 after a period of several years working as the resident psychologist at Parramatta Prison. During that time I had established a number of world-leading programmes, including a scheme for juvenile offenders whereby they spent the day in prison at Parramatta to deter them from a future life of crime. The programme involved them living the day as a prisoner with being exposed to the process of being locked in a prison cell over lunch and eating the gruel, which is standard prison food. In the afternoon they reported to four trained prisoners who would explain the realities of prison life in the context of their own commensurate with juvenile crime, which more often than not eventually led to them serving sentences in excess of 30 years for murder. Because of this programme, I was invited to provide an address at the inaugural congress to the Australian and New Zealand Association of Psychiatry, Psychology and Law. Much to the chagrin of my colleagues and older practitioners, my talk captured the imagination of the Melbourne press, with me being pictured on the front page of The Melbourne Age *on the following Monday morning. It was at this conference that I had the very good fortune to meet my business partner-to-be, the late Dr. David Sime. He was evidently impressed by my potential and suggested that it would not harm my career in the least if I relocated to Melbourne and worked with him.*

I was 27 years of age at the time and while highly flattered, I surprised him by saying that I preferred my Balmain lifestyle, embracing as it did numerous hotels, beaches and women. Sime, however, was more stubborn and resilient than I had anticipated. To this end he somewhat arrogantly commenced referring me work from Melbourne, with him contacting me and stating in his nonchalant voice, "I hope you don't mind, Tim, but I have booked four people for you to see this coming Saturday...I have organized for you to use my room and I shall collect you at the airport on Friday night". The deal was done when he indeed collected me in his brand new Mercedes and advised that if I worked in Melbourne, I could buy one of my own within 12 months. Sime was true to his word and in the weekend that I worked in Melbourne in early 1981, I earned more than I was taking home each month from the prison. Because of this, I agreed to try Melbourne for a year.

Sime and I were involved in establishing the first trauma debriefing company in Australia when we approached a number of banks to propose a more effective and efficient way to deal with their staff in the wake of armed hold-ups. This involved a "ghost busters" approach whereby we would have a counsellor present at a bank branch that had been robbed within an hour of the event. We commenced with the ANZ Bank, which was our first robbery at Preston in 1985. By the end of that year, we had acquired all of the bank's names including the NAB, Westpac and the Commonwealth Bank and had established offices in each of the capital cities. To service our model, we employed in excess of 30 psychologists around the country on a sub-contracting basis.

In addition, I had the privilege of being retained as a Visiting Fellow and an Advisory Board Member at Melbourne University, and the honour of being voted the National Chairman of the College of Forensic Psychologists within the Australian Psychological Society. The cigars and cash were rolling in by the truck load. As the scheme gained greater notoriety, invitations to address international conferences beckoned and as a consequence my fame as a psychologist escalated. While this business continued, so too did my forensic practice against a backdrop as a young man in his mid-30s believing that he was invincible and being seduced by his own bullshit.

Little wonder then that I was the last to recognize the serious steps of my depressive illness. I had some inkling that all was not well during 1997 when my sense of humour dissipated and I was becoming, according to my partner, increasingly irritable and difficult to live with. I was clearly running out of steam but lacked the insight to recognize the connection between this and the very nature of the work I was doing.

Forensic psychology is not for the fainthearted, both in terms of the content of the work and the extraordinary pressures which can be brought to bear as an expert witness under cross-examination. Although my reputation had always been very positive in terms of my capacity to equip myself in court, it was nonetheless due that with the effluxion of time I was becoming increasingly worn out. It was in this context that in my early 40s, after having never abused drugs in the past, I foolishly agreed to sample a line of cocaine which had been offered to me at a Melbourne luncheon for a number of leading legal practitioners. I found the impact of cocaine immediately seductive and powerful with this having the effect of energizing me and offsetting my sense of depression. For some time beforehand, I had been plagued with recurring thoughts regarding the Hoddle Street massacre, as in the enthusiasm of a young practitioner I had immersed myself in what was the biggest criminal case in the country. This involved not only interviewing the accused over a 12-month period but also being privy to much of the forensic evidence which included photographs of the cadavers of his victims. These were horrific and I noticed, although a considerable period of time had lapsed, that I was having continuous flashbacks to these images and thinking about the families of the deceased. It may well have been that it was 10 years after the event that my unconscious mind broke through the surface of consciousness.

In any event, I found that my first try of cocaine liberated me from these feelings. In this context, in retrospect it was of no surprise that with ongoing time occasional usage became a well-entrenched habit to the point of addiction. This process was galvanized by the diagnosis of my wife's illness and my attempts to maintain emotional and physical support for her and our children as well as running an exceptionally busy practice.

All of this came to a crashing halt on 9/11, 1999 and in the ensuing days when I volunteered myself forward to the Victorian Police at St. Kilda Road. I was beyond my elastic limits and felt the only way to move forward was to come clean. I had a clear choice to entirely change my life or to remain forever wallowing in the sewer which I had created for myself. My concern and love for my family provided no alternative other than to move forward with my rehabilitation and recovery.

In retrospect, after years of self-reflection I can appreciate how naïve I was to assume that simply by making a decision to cease using cocaine within a matter of weeks my judgment, cognition and mood would improve. There are a number of other further life events which mitigated against this, including not only the death of my first wife three weeks beforehand but in addition the death of my *much-loved business partner of over 20 years, David Sime. He died suddenly from a heart attack three weeks to the day following surrendering myself to the police. I was then faced with the additional ignominy of having to face court in December 1999, where fortunately I encountered a sympathetic magistrate who stated on the record "that my integrity was beyond reproach". In this context I was given a good behaviour bond without a conviction on the basis of him adding that he did not wish to interfere in any way in what had been a very significant career. I thought that this would be the end of my woes and heralded a new beginning in terms of my recovery. I was sadly mistaken, however, in not recognizing the power of the former Psychologists Registration Board of Victoria with whom I had previously locked horns, who in their collective wisdom decided to hold an inquiry into my fitness and ability to practice.*

Once I received a letter requesting my presence before the Board, I realized I was doomed. The proceedings continued for a period of six months during which numerous character witnesses were called on my behalf, including a County Court Judge and a range of top Melbourne QCs representing the literati of the profession, with one person stating that my addiction had come as a great shock to them as it had never been reflected in the quality of my work.

June 20th, 2000 was my second 9/11. This was the day when I was formally deregistered, although by this stage, despite the considerable press attention in my case, my practice had recovered and I had then been drug-free in excess of eight months.

Sadly, however, despite the best efforts of the QC representing me, I was stripped of my right to practice. The timing of this decision was exquisite, if not curious, having by that stage been free of drugs in excess of nine months and being well on the way to recovery through psychotherapy and medication. I was hence left in the unenviable position of having my reputation and career shattered, dealing with unresolved grief from the death of my first wife, and having to care for five children, including my newborn son who was at that stage eight months of age. The hypocrisy of this decision was recently reflected in an article referring to drugs in sport and a series of quotations from members of the Australian Psychological Society, who essentially stated that sportsmen using drugs should not be deprived of their career, as the loss of identity associated with being unable to continue in employment is a major obstacle and hurdle to recovering. It would consequently appear that with the effluxion of some 14 years, greater insight to this obvious course of action has occurred. Well done!

I have never been known to be one who wallows in self-pity and in this context I had only one realistic path ahead of me, which was to continue with my recovery and to re-enter the workforce in some capacity. Friends suggested that I should publish a book concerning my career and my very public downfall. I was put in contact with a publisher at Random House and commenced work. In addition, I was contacted by a close friend, Professor Paul Wilson, who was Dean of the Humanities Faculty at Bond University. Because of the considerable media attention that my case had attracted, Paul as a true friend offered immense support, among many others within the legal profession. Professor Wilson, in conjunction with another very close friend, Assistant Professor John Ritchie (PhD), invited me to give a public lecture at Bond University. Following this I was offered a position as an Adjunct Visiting Professor and a seat on the Advisory Board to the Department's School of Applied Psychology and Criminology. This opportunity represented a major step forward in my recovery as I felt that notwithstanding what had occurred, at least some people who mattered at a professional level had sufficient faith and trust in me to overcome my difficulties. To this day, I cannot sufficiently express my gratitude to both Paul and John for giving me the platform to relaunch my life. This vital platform enabled me to relaunch my self-esteem and consequently my professional life.

Cocaine is a stimulant drug, which acts in many and varied insidious ways. Because of its neurological impact and, in particular, its working by releasing large quantities of dopamine neurotransmitters associated with reward, the process of addiction is rapid. This knowledge that was acquired through considerable reading on the topic, coupled with discussions with experts in the field, gave me some understanding as to why my personality and behaviour had changed so dramatically within such a brief period of time.

At another level, it suppresses appetite. As a consequence, I lost a significant quantity of weight during the period of my abuse, and upon cessation I rapidly gained in excess of 20 kilograms. This clearly reflects the deleterious impact of the drug on one's physical health. Because of the weight gain my self-esteem, which was already at rock bottom, was further affected. I was transformed from a previously confident and articulate individual to one who struggled on a daily basis, despairing that the best days of my life had already been experienced and that my future was bleak.

Due to my recovering judgment I realized that however severe my depression was, I needed to persevere with physical exercise.

One cannot overstate the importance of regular exercise in terms of maintaining psychological equilibrium in the context of stressing the body, leading to the release of endorphins which enhance mood. There is well-established research concerning the fact that exercise is a natural prophylactic against depression and anxiety. Beyond speaking to a mental health practitioner, for the first time in my life I exposed my insecurities with trusted friends. I was greatly assisted in my recovery by the love and support of my second wife, Carla Lechner, who is a highly regarded clinical and forensic psychologist. My mood, however, was infiltrated by all-pervasive feelings of guilt concerning not just my behaviour but the substantial impact which this had had upon those that I love most. Due to the loss of income and my rapid transformation from "rooster to feather duster", the situation of our household would change from one of affluence to financial struggle. Against this backdrop, I found myself selling my loved artwork and antiques as well as our home in order to survive.

In retrospect, this "trial by ordeal" clearly strengthened my character and ironically made me realize for the first time that the perception of my ability in the community was not a new artefact but, in fact, I possessed the inner strength to deal with major catastrophe. The support and love from my family and others including random letters I received from people in the community supporting my position was what helped me to survive the darkest period in my life.

Recovery from major depression and addiction is a slow process. I had initially and naïvely assumed that by ceasing drug use my mental equilibrium would within a matter of days, if not weeks, bounce back to normal. This could not have been further from the truth. Every day I was plagued with self-doubt, self-recrimination and despair regarding my future. I could not believe that I had obliterated such a stellar career with such majestic stupidity. There were many times when I felt that it was "all too hard" and it would be fair to say that the thought of ending my life on occasions filtered into my consciousness. Once again, however, the reality check of the impact of this upon my family and those who believed in me pulled me back. In addition to ongoing psychotherapy, which at one point involved seeing a practitioner twice a week to unload the considerable emotional detritus of my former life, I maintained exercise and attempted as best I could to overcome my black thoughts.

During this period of rehabilitation, my marriage became understandably very strained. Carla was furious with me and rightly so, although at the time I was so filled with my own despair and anger that I could not fully appreciate the dimension of hers. It is perhaps a very real example of the importance of marriage vow referable to supporting one another for better, for worse, for richer, for poorer, in sickness and in health, that for the sake of our beautiful children, who had already suffered enough, we persevered with our issues and ultimately worked through them. Despite this, however, I was plagued with insecurity and self-doubt, which was augmented by the humiliation and financial castration I had suffered due to the loss of my right to work as a professional.

Addiction is very much a disease of loneliness, and in this context, through the effluxion of time, it became increasingly apparent to me that in large measure, I had formed a relationship with this drug to offset my feelings of isolation and self-doubt. Consequently I needed to fully effect a positive trajectory to establish new friendships and re-engage former friends who maintained a positive and healthy lifestyle. I was amazed by the substantial support which I received from all whom I approached.

Some 18 months after losing my Practising Certificate, on advice from a number of eminent lawyers, I made the decision to apply for re-registration. This hearing lasted for a brief time and I sensed even before it had concluded that my pleas of self-recovery were falling on deaf ears. This was the case with me once again being subjected to a humiliating decision that I was still not an individual of good character. Fortunately, however, by this time I had recovered sufficiently to not allow this view to destroy the positive work I had done in terms of getting back on my feet. In this context, I resolved to continue working on the issues in the firm belief that however long it took, ultimately I would regain my Practising Certificate.

As it eventuated, after three and a half years which in reality felt like a lifetime, I represented myself once again before the Board and was re-admitted to practice. There were, however, caveats placed upon this, including me receiving professional supervision for two years, which I was happy to embrace in terms of further developing my knowledge. More importantly, it represented a small step in a long journey to a fuller recovery.

Despite this very positive development, I nonetheless feared that I may well have won the battle but lost the war against the backdrop of my concerns that my standing had been so severely damaged that no legal practitioner would be prepared to take the risk to refer cases to me. Nothing could have been further from the truth, and I was greeted by former professional colleagues in the legal fraternity as a long-lost friend.

At the time of putting pen to paper, it has now been nearly eight years since I have returned to work. Initially the referral rate was very slow and in large measure the household survived at a financial level through Carla's prodigious work ethic. This was both in terms of developing her own private practice in Melbourne, as well as caring for our children and indeed me. It took a number of years before I began to feel confident that both my self-employment and financial viability could be maintained.

Life teaches us many lessons. Although I would not wish the process which I endured during this Felliniesque phase of my career on anyone else, I have come out of the darkness a much more humble and paradoxically stronger person. I have endeavoured to use the lessons which I have learned in terms of recovery from drug abuse, depression, anxiety and so on to assist the numerous people who are now referred to me for forensic assessment. Although I was initially ashamed about my prior drug use, I now use my recovery as a working example to others that no matter how harsh a blow life may deal you, it is always possible with perseverance, love and support, and a willingness to open oneself to others, to recover.

I am now extraordinarily busy once again working in Melbourne, Sydney and the Northern parts of New South Wales, although unlike in the past, I have managed to establish a solid work/lifestyle balance. To this end, I am fully aware of the warning signs of burnout and stress and when they appear on the horizon, I cut back on my commitments. I nonetheless fight on a daily basis *a tendency towards workaholism and I still seek counsel from professional people and friends in terms of this particular issue. Although it is a struggle, I still endeavour to maintain a degree of physical fitness. I also regularly receive vitamin shots, adopting a holistic and committed approach to maintaining well-being. The fact that I have been able to resurrect my career has finally, at the age of 58, made me realize that perhaps after all my early success was not a fluke. It was a reflection of an innate capacity which, had it not been for this major crisis in my life, I may never have realized truly existed.*

Addiction in Business

Why do we read so many stories about high-flying, successful people in business, politics and entertainment falling from peaks of influence and social standing? They often lose it all and in many cases end up bankrupt and sometimes in jail which, for intelligent people, seems to make no sense at all. The media is constantly featuring stories of highly successful people completely losing everything. These people have previously demonstrated an obvious high level of discipline, intelligence, awareness and tenacity to build a huge career in business and commerce only to inexplicably self-implode.

I think in most cases the reason why this happens, usually around the mid-life crisis years, is very much intertwined with addiction. The very reason why certain men became successful is due in the first place to their addictive personalities. Success doesn't happen by chance, and these men needed various qualities in order to succeed. But it is worth questioning whether addiction played a part in that success as well as in their eventual downfall. In reading biographies of successful people (Ted Turner being an example), it's often not a great surprise to find depression being a factor in their drive for success.

Success provides us with a lot of leeway to indulge and therefore impair our judgment. When you have plenty of fame and money, the indulgences can become more obscured and somehow it seems "OK" to partake in drugs, prostitution and other illegal acts. Moreover, society seems to accept this because these men are famous. Very few street junkies taking cocaine end up in the glossy magazines or have people throwing money at them. Perhaps this is another form of mid-life crisis when we suddenly realize most of our important aims in life have been achieved. The thrill of the rise and the excitement of achieving new things are replaced by a feeling of nothing left to do.

I know a number of wealthy, highly successful men who all seem to have suffered from feelings of emptiness later in life. They have achieved enormous success and wealth and have everything materially that most men would want. Yet while they may not have imploded completely, they are filled with a hollow feeling that the best things of life are already over. Quite often depression plays a key factor in their lives as the high level of excitement enjoyed on the way up is simply no longer there. They are in search of something which becomes ever more elusive.

Another key influence is the simple fact that while these men have spent their lives working long hours, being totally devoted to building their business empires and careers, they have done it at the expense of their health. In many cases, they are prematurely aged and are unable to enjoy their success or wealth. This is a more common situation than most people understand and may explain why we are hearing so many tragic stories of downfalls in the press.

The former head of the International Monetary Fund (IMF) was so clearly addicted to certain sexual exploits that he completely destroyed his chances of becoming President of France. And did Bernie Madoff, the famous Ponzi scheme embezzler, really just get carried away (as he claimed) or possibly did he have an addiction to the wealth and social standing that he enjoyed? Was he possibly addicted to the constant risk he lived with every day?

I think the simple fact is that no matter where a man stands in life, if he has an addictive personality, the time will come when he can lose all normal and moral values. This is especially true if he has not looked after his body and shows the signs of premature ageing. This problem among men in business, political life and many other sectors may well be endemic. The fact that someone is rich and powerful doesn't stop them from experiencing the emptiness that the years ahead can bring. This is the simple old-fashioned, mid-life crisis.

Ten tips to help you deal with addiction:

1. We all have addictions.
2. It gets worse as you get older.
3. It's never too late to admit you have a problem.
4. Admit to yourself you have a problem first.
5. Then, admit to someone else you have a problem.
6. Feel relieved when you do seek help.
7. Those close to you get hurt the most.
8. Some addictive behaviour can have positive components.
9. Those close to you already know – it's no big secret.
10. You can lose everything if you don't stop.

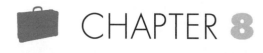

CHAPTER 8

LOVE DRUGS

Secrets to get your sex life back on track

Well, wouldn't it be wonderful if there was a drug that could help us love better and be better lovers? I know if I had access to such a drug, I would quite happily be the human guinea pig. What man wouldn't take such a potion?

In reality, men's roles have become so morphed and confused in recent years, it's become difficult to find our place in the whole mix. And as we get older, we only get more confused. Men in their 40s and 50s today effectively bring values and perceptions of their role as men from a different era – the era of their parents and especially their fathers, which are no longer relevant. This is no more apparent than when it comes to love.

We are now older and in most cases a little scarred from the disappointments and let-downs experienced previously. This is the stage of life at which we can take one of two directions, whether that's in an existing relationship or looking for a new one. For the age-nostic man, that direction is one which sees him maintaining his energy, belief and, most importantly, his hope that love has not left his life for good and that it is still within the realms of possibility. It is all to do with the belief that it is not behind you but all ahead of you.

I am writing this piece in Los Angeles and last night I had dinner with a friend who, while he has a brilliant Hollywood career and is reaching the pinnacle of that, was coming out of a difficult relationship break-up and at 48 years of age was battling with the belief that maybe it had all passed him by.

We had a long conversation about the subject of love and what it meant to him. I tried very hard to keep the conversation positive as he was hurting and was feeling defeated. Basically, he is a good-looking, highly intelligent man, who clearly has a good heart. But he was overweight and that wonderful sense of humour was now only lurking in the shadows. He was also now drinking a little too much as a means of self-medication and was lacking in confidence. I was really feeling for him and quite frankly he was the perfect reader for this book.

We had last met a few months ago and he mentioned he had never forgotten our last conversation about what I had chosen to do in order to rejuvenate myself. I told him I couldn't understand why all men weren't doing it. He laughed and said, "Well, it's all right for you. You are 53 and look and act 33!" I simply said, "Exactly! That's the way I have decided to age."

We got back to the delicate subject of love, and I told him that if he wanted to find love again, he had to get back on track. He didn't have to become some "new man"; he just had to get back to being the man he was when he was 35. Quite simply, to be attractive to the opposite sex, you have to portray youth, energy and health.

I had a discussion with a cosmetic surgeon only that day on what attractiveness in men really meant. As a cosmetic surgeon with many years' experience, he was convinced about the answer: you don't have to be good-looking as a man; the main component of attractiveness in men was having a look of energy, youth and health. The worst look is one of tiredness. Subliminally, nothing more will turn a woman off than a tired-looking man. It is primal, apparently, because subconsciously as a man you want to show her that you can protect and take care of her – the number one thing most women want.

Looking younger – having great skin, a youthful face and a fit body – helps, but this is not the main component of attractiveness in men for women.

So before we get onto the so-called "love drugs", my first advice to you guys is to get the BASICS right. Look the best you can, lose the extra weight, drop the old-man attitude, walk with a youthful spring and portray a playful attitude to life. This is the age-nostic man at his best and will give you a great chance of keeping or finding love again.

And if you can't get the basics right and all else fails, get some good shoes. Apparently many women judge men by their shoes. So if you are prematurely fat and walking and talking like an old man, then just have incredible shoes on at all times, even in bed! And for heaven's sake, have a sense of humour – this is the biggest thing we lose as men as we get older. We lose our lightness and playfulness and become far too serious. Lighten up! Now for the secrets that will help.

The Reality

First, let's admit that our sex life just ain't what it used to be unless you started having sex for the first time at the age of 40, which is highly unlikely. The fact of the matter is our bodies simply don't perform how they did when we were younger. We all remember our 20s and 30s when sex was all we could think about, and I am sure if we had put the same amount of effort into other areas of our lives, we would all be ruling the world or at least some large corporation by now. Even though we may not be able to perform at such a high level, it doesn't mean we shouldn't have a fun and highly rewarding sex life.

It is a biological fact that most of us experience lowering levels of hormone in our bodies as we age. This has many impacts but does make us more prone to depression and lack of energy. This is something which can so easily affect our sex drive and, as a result, a growing number of people now turn to hormone replacement therapy (HRT) to help them. This whole area of medicine has had a rather dark cloud hanging over it and is seen by many as being "not natural". The reality is that we can get our bodies feeling younger in any area, which affects so many other parts of our health and well-being.

There are other factors that contribute to lower sex drive and the urge for physical intimacy. Our lives simply get more serious and, in many cases, we have families, mortgages, children, large credit card bills, careers and many other responsibilities. After a hard day, the overwhelming feeling when we drag ourselves onto that comfortable bed is rest, not more activity. My view is that we have to fight this feeling whenever possible because sex is important, not just for the health of our relationships but also to maintain our own body. Our DNA includes a need to continue having sex, which keeps us more in tune with our feelings and behaviour as we get older.

Just as important a contributor to a declining sex life is that we simply don't look as good as we did. Our waistlines are often larger and we don't feel as virile or ready for considerable sexual exertion. We are also bombarded with magazines, advertisements and plenty of other media of young fit men who only remind us of our past, not where we are today. We should all have to watch a video of the first years together with our partners and how our sex life was back then. Let's face it, very few couples ever decide to get together because their sex life was totally rubbish and they wanted to spend a lousy life together by getting married. Somehow as we get older, we seem to place far more importance on other aspects of our life and place our sex life on the back-burner. I believe this has been a major contributory factor in divorce rates, the rise of depression and less happiness in society.

The Good News

So that's the depressing part for most of us, but there is plenty we can do to avoid this seemingly inevitable slide. First, whether we are in a relationship or not, it's time to take a good look at ourselves. So strip down to nothing, get a paper bag over your head and put two holes in it so you can see yourself in the mirror. Have a good look because that is who you are and what your partner or prospective partner sees. This might come as a surprise but your partner really doesn't find a somewhat bulging belly, flabby arms or jowly face all that sexy, especially when you are on top of her!

She loves you and still wants to have sex with you but if you really want it to be the best possible experience, you need to make a concerted effort because if you don't, it is only going to get worse. The further down this road toward obesity you go, the tougher it will be to turn around and walk in the other direction. If you don't take an interest in your body, why should your partner? Having confidence in your own shape also helps you look and act more positive, something that women usually notice far quicker than us guys.

I have blamed us men for letting ourselves go but our other halves also have some responsibility. Have you ever noticed that a lot of obese people seem to be obese as a couple? It is almost like they have looked at each other and agreed that if one was going to get fat and unattractive, then so will the other. I call them "fat couples". It almost looks like a competition. Next time you are at an airport or shopping centre, have a look around and you will see there are a lot of fat couples all competing to be unattractive for each other. In the same vein you will see slim, fit and healthy couples together also. Subconsciously many seem to have turned into role models for each other.

Getting It Up

It is unbelievable to think that approximately 30 million men are affected by erectile dysfunction (ED) in the United States alone. According to the NHS in the UK, it is estimated that 50% of men between 40 and 70 years of age will experience ED at least once. If a man cannot achieve or maintain an erection, it causes feelings of inadequacy, frustration, self-doubt, low confidence and low self-esteem. We've all experienced it but blame the alcohol or the situation. It is terrible when it happens! It's a subject which few men like to discuss openly, but I did manage to have a man-to-man conversation with Dr. Michael Zacharia and discuss the intricacies of ED and what can be done about it.

Michael Hogg: *Just how common is it? Are we men facing a crisis?*
Michael Zacharia: Almost all of my male friends in their 30s and above have had some sort of erectile dysfunction. Give them a drink or two and it sky-rockets dramatically again. How many times have I been asked for prescriptions for Viagra or Cialis? Plenty! The number of guys I know who boast to their mates of their bedroom capabilities, but come and ask me for a little help, "just to make their partner happy", occurs more often than I can remember.

MH: *So why does ED occur?*
MZ: There are certain risk factors, all of which affect blood flow through the body but particularly may reduce blood flow in the penis. These include high blood pressure, abnormally high blood lipids, obesity, diabetes and smoking. And let's not forget mood swings, depression and the use of anti-depressants. While it is fairly well established that testosterone plays a role in libido or sexual desire, its precise contribution to erectile function remains unclear. So if you are fat, depressed, smoke, don't exercise and have a low testosterone level, you are likely to have a problem getting it up.

MH: *So what is ED exactly?*
MZ: It is the inability to have an erection or maintain an erection. It can happen at any age but there is no doubt it occurs more commonly as we get

older. Young guys usually have no problem with achieving an erection and maintaining it, and even having another erection soon after climaxing. As we get older and an erection eventually comes along, it will usually take a lot longer to come again. The other issue, of course, is premature ejaculation, which can affect all ages. This may occur more commonly in younger men and can be embarrassing and humiliating in some cases!

It is not too far from the truth when the opposite sex state that a man's brain is in his penis. An erection actually begins in the brain and is largely under the control of the central nervous system (CNS). Physical and mental stimulation cause nerves from the brain to send signals and chemical messages to nerves in the penis, which allow the penile blood vessels to relax and hence blood flows into the penis. These tissues that fill are known as corpus cavernosum and corpus spongiosum. Once the blood engorges these tissues, the high pressure traps the blood (like a rubber band closing off the exit) and maintains the erection.

During sexual stimulation, the brain sends signals that result in the release of nitric oxide by parasympathetic nerves in the penis. An enzyme called cyclic guanosine monophosphate (cGMP) is released and prompts the smooth muscles of penile arteries to relax, allowing more blood to flow into the spongy tissues of the penis. Simultaneously, blood return via penile veins is restricted, trapping blood in the organ, resulting in engorgement and erection. Eventually, cGMP is broken down by an enzyme Phosphodiesterase 5 (PDE5) and when this occurs, the erection subsides; blood flow returns to normal, and the penis resumes its normal flaccid state.

MH: *And how can we go about treating ED?*
MZ: The chain of events leading to erection presents several opportunities for intervention in the treatment of ED. Increasing the availability of nitric oxide is one, while decreasing the activity of PDE5 is another. Viagra, Cialis and Levitra, for instance, are selective inhibitors of PDE5. By inhibiting the degradation of cGMP, which is the direct intracellular mediator of the nitric oxide pathway, these drugs promote better erections – but not without side effects and risks. Viagra may temporarily affect colour vision and in rare cases may cause blindness, but the most common problem is headache or

facial flushing, a blocked nose or nausea. Any of these drugs may induce a sustained erection that does not subside after more than four hours – a potentially damaging condition known as priapism.

MH: *The subject of premature ejaculation is on most men's minds (and women's).*
MZ: We don't know exactly why PE occurs but when it does it can be just as embarrassing as not being able to get it up. Ejaculation is triggered when we reach a critical level of excitement. Sexual stimulation causes nerves in the penis to send chemical messages or impulses to the spinal cord and into the brain where other chemical messages are sent back to the penis – via the spinal cord – causing ejaculation.

Ejaculation has two phases. During the first phase, the vas deferens, which are the tubes that store and transport sperm from the testes, contract to squeeze sperm toward the back of the urethra. The seminal vesicles also release secretions into the back of the urethra. During the second phase, the posterior urethra senses the secretions within it (at the height of sexual excitement) and sends signals to the spinal cord. In turn, it sends powerful signals to the muscles at the base of penis to vigorously contract every 0.8 seconds and force the semen out of the penis. The only way we can delay ejaculation is to "train" the penis by pulling out and removing stimulus, waiting, then going for it again. Also, the more a man has sex, it seems the longer he can go. The only medication that seems to delay ejaculation is low doses of an anti-depressant called Clomipramine. This has been combined with my mate Dr. Jack's wafers and it seems to work.

MH: *Do supplements really work to enhance erectile function?*
MZ: Some supplements will improve ED by increasing testosterone levels, but others act directly on the penile tissue. The supplements that increase testosterone seem to inhibit the activity of aromatase, the enzyme that facilitates the transformation of testosterone into oestrogen, thereby increasing levels. Grape Seed Extract, Resveratrol, Chrysin and Zinc are all supplements that can do this. Other supplements that may have a direct effect on ED include arginine, Bulgarian tribulus, yohimbine, gingko and icariin. Arginine is an amino acid the body uses to produce nitric oxide (NO).

We know NO relaxes smooth muscle in the penis and allows an increase in blood flow in many parts of the body including the penis.

Noradrenaline is the principal neurotransmitter that causes the smooth blood vessels in the penile arteries to contract and end an erection. Yohimbine (also known as yohimbe) is derived from the bark of an African evergreen tree. It blocks brain receptors involved in releasing noradrenaline in the genitals and so has the effect of improving erections. In some countries, Yohimbine requires a prescription because it has a direct effect on the brain rather than the penis. Icariin, ginko and tribulus also all in their own way enhance erectile function.

Most of us need to lose weight and get fitter. But assuming you are willing to do that, there are some other things the age-nostic man can do to enhance his sex life and that of his partner. There is no doubt that as we age, we do need some help from time to time. Our lives are busy, often stressful and, at times, we can feel low. This is often a result of our lower hormone levels rather than our lifestyles, but the two are usually heavily inter-related.

Earlier, we discussed hormones and hormone replacement (in Chapter 4). There are two chemicals we generate naturally – hormone and testosterone – and both have a huge effect on our sex lives, especially after the age of 40. I am no doctor, but there are two areas in our sex lives that are relatively simple to explain. One is desire or libido and the other is performance. There are a number of easy-to-purchase products out there that can make a huge difference in both these areas.

Enhancers

I have always believed that natural products are best. However, on some occasions a pharmaceutical product is needed, such as Viagra and Cialis. These don't cure the problem but can provide a short-term lift. Attacking the root causes of sex drive is the only meaningful solution.

I have had many discussions about these products and the question I always hear is, "Why does one need to take them?" The answer is, you may not need them but they do help. Both products are excellent as an enhancer to sex, especially when one is tired or stressed. These simple little pills give us that edge to perform at our best and when we really think about it, they are really used for our partner's pleasure, not our own. So they are one of the rare unselfish things we men can do in our sex lives. But there is not much point taking them in the first place if we don't have the desire for sex and that is often the big problem for us as we age.

Testosterone

I am a big proponent of testosterone replacement therapy due to its positive effect on our sex lives as we age. I have been on testosterone replacement since 2008 and I know what a difference it makes to my libido, not to mention all the other benefits to my mood and energy. It's no coincidence that the three pillars of age-nostic medicine (mood, energy and vitality) are at a peak in our 20s and early 30s. Let's face it, we don't meet many 20-year-old men with lousy sex lives who are depressed and have no energy. If you do, it's normally because they have been abusing themselves with other stimulants and/or have a lifestyle that brings on such a state.

I will say as a non-medical person, it is my belief that testosterone replacement is the most important single thing a man can do if he is going to lead a truly age-nostic lifestyle. It is all about getting our levels in balance with sensible replacement (not abuse).

Why is testosterone important? Well, testosterone is a steroid hormone. In men, it plays a key role in the development of reproductive tissues as well as influencing other sexual characteristics such as increased muscle and bone density, which directly relates to our strength. In addition, testosterone is essential for health and well-being as it helps the prevention of osteoporosis. On average, in adult males, the plasma concentration of testosterone is about 7-8 times greater than the concentration of adult females, but as the metabolic consumption of testosterone in males is greater, the daily production is about 20 times greater in men. Testosterone is observed in most vertebrates, which are key to our flexibility and mobility. Lower levels of testosterone can also lead to issues relating to cholesterol and glycemic control.

What is important about testosterone is not just that it gives us our sex drive but that it also affects many other things in our body and mind.

Higher levels of testosterone are usually associated with periods of sexual activity. This is fairly obvious, but what it means is that if we have less sex, our testosterone levels start to fall. This makes it doubly difficult to get things back on track should we have a period of low or no sex. One thing probably not to tell your partner is men who have sexual encounters with unfamiliar or multiple partners experience larger increases of testosterone the morning after. If we were to watch a sexually explicit movie, we are likely to have an above average increase in testosterone, peaking well after the end of the film. Some research has shown that men who watch explicit films also report increased optimism and decreased exhaustion. This shows how important this balance is for our bodies. Testosterone increases in men who engage in brief conversations with women they find attractive. That's another good excuse for chatting to pretty girls as often as you can! But seriously, we should be switched on to how our levels of testosterone vary and what we can do to improve them.

We are all aware of some of the physical impacts of having more of this natural wonder drug running round our body, but it also creates a substantial impact on our mind. As testosterone affects the entire body, so the brain is also affected. Much of the literature I have read over the last 10 years suggests that attention, memory and spatial ability are key functions affected by testosterone. These are core building blocks for performance in the office as well as the bedroom. By upping our levels of testosterone, we can improve our mental capability in several ways, helping us compete with the younger guys and making us feel a whole lot better at the same time.

Oxytocin

When we talk about so-called "love drugs", oxytocin usually comes immediately to the forefront. It is the ultimate hormone when it comes to love and bonding between two people.

Oxytocin is a hormone mainly given off when a woman is in labour and when she is breast feeding. It also occurs when you have an orgasm. It is called the bonding hormone for good reason. As we get older, especially after 40, we lose a lot of our ability to be close to others, especially if we are in a relationship. A lot of this could be due to the loss of this special hormone. Research in this area is still going on, but there are a number of interesting articles available about oxytocin and the effect it has on us, which you can find on the Internet.

Of all the supplements mentioned in this book, oxytocin seems to produce the most interest, especially from women, who in most cases want to obtain it in order to give it to their partners. It has been well documented through research that taking oxytocin will intensify orgasms, especially for women. But studies also show that even holding hands or hugging someone will naturally increase oxytocin levels in both sexes. Oxytocin also appears to make you more trusting and willing to bond (or re-bond) with people close to you and this seems to be the most profound benefit of taking it on a regular basis.

In terms of negative effects shown by studies, taking oxytocin can make you too trusting and possibly bond with people on a deeper level than you would normally do. I can only say that having taken this supplement for over a year, I have never experienced this "side effect". Friends of mine who have given oxytocin to their partners have noticed a definite positive change in their response to them. And the partners themselves have noticed the effect in themselves.

Oxytocin is known as the "love hormone". Some research suggests that taking oxytocin will make you more attractive to the opposite sex. But of course that will only happen if you have all the other elements under control (i.e. keeping yourself in the best possible shape both physically and mentally). I have no doubt that taking oxytocin regularly does make you more attractive in the sense that you are more open and warm as a person and more willing to bond with someone. As you get older, and have been scarred by past disappointments with love and lost the ability to trust easily, oxytocin can help you overcome those challenges and become more confident and positive as you seek better or new relationships.

So, by now, you are probably wondering how you can get started on your own age-nostic journey. This depends on which country you are in and when you are reading this book. To begin your next chapter, visit www. genagenostic.com. Most clinics that specialize in anti-ageing for men view oxytocin as an excellent age-nostic supplement, with huge benefits for men, and will have oxytocin available.

The Backbone to the Age-nostic Regime

In summary, testosterone and oxytocin will usually form a significant part of any age-nostic programme. But before including them in yours, you must consult your doctor and get your blood tested in order to check your testosterone levels and your PSA (which is the blood test marker for any problems that may be identified with your prostate, especially if you are over 50).

There is no doubt in my mind that testosterone replacement treatment can transform your life in many ways besides your sex life. Your mood and well-being in general will be enhanced and that grumpy old man feeling will soon disappear. You will invigorate the youth that you feel you are losing or have already lost. Of course, you will have to try it for yourself and experience the benefits before being totally convinced of it. But I am now in the fourth year of my testosterone replacement treatment, and while I do many of the other things outlined in this book, I strongly believe that testosterone has become the backbone of my age-nostic regime. Most likely, I will continue having it for the rest of my life, even past my 100th birthday!

As for oxytocin, well, I do take it regularly, but often I take breaks from it for a week or two. Even if it is just a placebo effect, which I strongly doubt, I still enjoy the results I experience with those around me. There are many other benefits from oxytocin, some of which may be real or not. For example, I was recently told that several high-flyers on Wall Street were taking oxytocin to become better at negotiating business deals and to come across as being more trusting and empathetic in those negotiations. Hopefully they are becoming more trusting and empathetic in their personal relationships and not just in business! In my mind, there is little doubt that the effects are real, and the benefits have been enormous from taking this supplement.

Ten tips to improve your sex life:

1. No one enjoys drunk sex.
2. If it's boring, don't blame her.
3. Do unto others as you would like others to do to you.
4. Sex starts outside the bedroom.
5. Don't be afraid of trying performance enhancers.
6. You don't have to perform like a 20-year-old, but you do need to try.
7. Nothing has really changed except that you have added some years.
8. Don't get tired or stale in your thoughts or actions.
9. If you make her laugh, you can make her come.
10. Slow it down and she will love you.

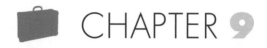

CHAPTER 9

FORMER FAT BAST**D

A common-sense approach to eating and dieting

These days when I telephone my friend Tim, I usually greet him by saying, "Hello former fat bast**d!" Tim has lost so much weight recently that the difference in him all round is quite amazing and so wonderful. It is heart-warming to see, as his life has truly changed in so many ways.

I am no expert, but when it comes to dieting and getting into shape, it is pretty simple: use your common sense. This is something I do more now as I am older than when I was younger – although the contradictions are always there. If I fall over, I always try and get back up, dust myself off and "have a meeting with myself" (as my mother used to say) before getting back on track. I believe the secret is not to keep going on a path that is clearly wrong and against what we know. This includes diets. We will fall over more as an adult man than we ever did as a toddler having just learned to walk – that's life.

So, if I was to write a bestselling diet book, it would have only one page, with the following advice:

"You know what to eat and what not to eat – just do it!"

And:

"Avoid anything with sugar in it."

The content of the biggest-selling diet book in history.

I mentioned Tim at the start of this chapter. Here is his personal account of his battle and eventual victory over his weight and diet problems. It is a truly inspirational story.

Addicted to Diets

By Tim Watson-Munro

During my secondary schooling, I had the great privilege of being sent to one of the finest establishments in Sydney renowned for its production of medical practitioners and members of the legal profession. It required an entrance exam to gain admission and my parents were understandably proud when I cut the mustard and was offered a place. I was reminded at a 40-year reunion a short time ago that I was best remembered not for my academic prowess but rather my ability on the sporting field. Indeed, in many ways, I chronically underachieved in the classroom as a result of boredom and laziness. When it came to sprinting and long jumping, however, my interest knew no boundaries. I had the privilege of representing my school at the GPS (Greater Public School) Finals and this no doubt established the platform for my healthy self-esteem in the ensuing years. Attendant to my capacity on the sports field and a rigorous programme of training which occupied most of my spare time, it would have been a challenge for an electronic microscope to find one micron of fat on my torso.

All of this changed as I left the prison service (resident psychologist at Parramatta Jail, Sydney) when I relocated to Melbourne to commence private practice in addition to taking on part-time academic work. The year was 1981, heralding the beginning of the gluttonous and greedy decade of the 80s. Around this time I was transformed from svelte athlete to Sir Lunch-a-Lot, as several days a week were spent enjoying long lunches after difficult court cases in the morning in an attempt to broaden my professional network. By this stage I was in my 30s, and by the end of the 80s I had bloomed from a lean 80 kilograms to approximately 90 kilograms in weight.

The mind can play wonderful tricks. Like "Mandrake, the Magician", it conjures up defence mechanisms to protect our egos against the reality in order to maintain some continuity in terms of one's sense of self. This occurred with me despite the obvious fact that I was becoming obese, with clear evidence of this in terms of my shirts no longer fitting and my suits needing refitting. I was nonetheless determined to believe that I was still the fit, young athlete that I recall during my teenage years and only slightly less so during my 20s.

In retrospect, my diet was atrocious with me consuming enormous amounts of calories each day in the form of rich fatty foods often washed down with fine red wine. Even the closest of my friends, who with the best of intentions would point to my protruding stomach in a derogatory fashion, could not budge this cognitive dissonance. Eventually I came to gather islets of insight, but reasoned that I was still young and had plenty of time to get rid of the weight if I chose to do so. Consequently the inevitable days of dieting and exercise were further forestalled.

One of the many insidious properties of cocaine is that it suppresses appetite to the point of virtual starvation. This is because it is a stimulant drug, which leads to vasoconstriction and the overloading of the adrenal system, which in turn has the effect of warding off hunger. This occurs at an unconscious level and only becomes apparent when the user, for the sake of social propriety, attempts to eat.

To illustrate the point, I recall vividly one episode during my stimulant abuse days where I was invited to a wedding. The reception was held at a well-known hotel in its private dining room where approximately 25 guests attended. The aperitifs prior to the main course involved a glass of champagne and a couple of lines of coke. Consequently, by the time the waiters began to serve the main meal, all patrons had lost their appetite and declined the food. It was extraordinary to see silver service trays with filet mignon, turkey and other delightful goodies being carried into our dining room only to be returned en masse. Certainly the chef, kitchen staff and waiters would have enjoyed a spectacular feast that evening. As my cocaine habit developed, my weight correspondingly fell off. By the time of my nadir in 1999, I had been on an unofficial Atkins Diet whereby all my fat reserves had been burnt beyond the minimal intake of protein and carbohydrates to the point where I had lost in the vicinity of 12 kilograms.

So dramatic was the change in my appearance that beyond losing two suit sizes, the same close friends who had cajoled me expressed concern that I may be suffering from a terminal illness. I looked emaciated and far from healthy. People would stop me in the street and ask with great concern, "Are you ok, Doc? You're looking very thin". None of these individuals were aware that I was struggling with my inner demons of addiction against a backdrop of attempting to maintain the façade of normalcy. Chinese whispers abound in all communities, and before too long I was receiving telephone calls from individuals whom I scarcely knew delicately enquiring as to whether I was dying.

When my cocaine use ceased in 1999 as abruptly as it had started a couple of years beforehand, my metabolism was thrown into disarray. It was as though the Formula One Ferrari, which had been driving my endocrine system and suppressing my weight, had blown up mid-track on the Ventura Highway and been replaced by an old jalopy. Indeed, my metabolism was zooming, and as a reaction to constant stress and not eating, it virtually stopped. Further compounding the problem of my retarded metabolism, for a time I "switched the bitch" and began drinking again on a fairly regular and at times heavy basis. I also resumed smoking after 20 years of cessation, which continued for about 12 months. This related to my high levels of anxiety regarding my future. Once my appetite was no longer suppressed, my weight rapidly returned. Within three months of ceasing drug use, I had gained approximately 20 kilograms in weight.

Since that time I have struggled to regain a healthy diet, lifestyle and weight loss. I experimented with the Atkins Diet only to find that my cholesterol levels sky-rocketed. It was reasonably effective but once I ceased, the weight returned. I tried other forms of diet, which provided only a temporary respite, with my weight then yo-yoing back. This in turn dented my self-esteem and began to affect my mood. I was becoming increasingly irritable and at a deeper level despairing that the best days were behind me, and I was destined for a life of obesity, coronary artery disease and in all likelihood, an early demise. Quite a shift from the sprint champion of the 1960s!

Galvanizing my despondency, my sleep deteriorated to the point where on more than one occasion I would awaken during the night to an empty bed with my wife having shifted to sleep on one of our children's bunk beds, as my snoring was overwhelming. Several years ago I travelled overseas with my family to visit my daughter who was on an exchange scholarship. We shared a three-bedroom suite with my family becoming increasingly hostile (bordering at times on hatred) as a consequence of my snoring, which they *allege had the same decibels as a freight train accelerating down a hill. I was oblivious to this and the associated health problems which my obesity and sleep disturbance was creating for my health until I was checked out by a physician, who advised in all likelihood that I was suffering from sleep apnoea. The evidence was incontrovertible and included dangerously high blood pressure and chronic fatigue during the day, which involved falling asleep at times and regular "nanna naps" on the weekends. I was still in a state of denial but eventually, with the cajoling of my family, I consented to have a sleep function test, which revealed that at frequent points during the night my blood oxygen content was dangerously low (60%). No wonder I was constantly tired, irritable and depressed.*

Sleep apnoea is the great undiagnosed health problem for men, and if left unchecked can lead to extremely serious consequences inclusive of stroke and heart attack, as well as industrial and motor vehicle accidents as a consequence of drowsiness and poor concentration. I was advised that I was having 74 apnoeic episodes per hour, which exceeded one per minute. Plainly speaking, this meant that my breathing was stopping on each occasion before my primitive brain restarted the process. When this was revealed I was filled with terror and panic, and immediately acquired a CPAP machine to rectify the problem. This, I reasoned, would also assist in me losing weight because I would sleep more effectively and consequently be more inclined to exercise.

Although the former occurred (I am now down to 0.04 apnoeic episodes an hour), my inclination for exercise failed to be resurrected. Compounding the problem, my family pointed out that I was constantly grazing when at home. Once again it ultimately became a situation of "mind over matter". In other words, you really have to be mentally focused as to what you eat, when you eat and how you eat (food mindfulness) to prevent the power of denial and rationalization overwhelming your motivation. When I commenced addressing my dietary issues, such as, for example, ceasing alcohol, I would then argue with my wife when she pointed out that I was drinking five large glasses of apple juice mixed with "diet" tonic water during the course of an evening. She correctly pointed out that I was essentially pouring sugar down my throat with me tersely responding, "I have given up booze and cheese, I deserve apple juice at least".

Another example related to my penchant for McDonald's food. I am constantly on the go in my professional life and find it very difficult to plan ahead in terms of my dietary requirements for the day. This takes effort and seems low on the priority list. In its absence, I would inevitably be seduced by the lure of the golden arches on the horizon, which intensified my hunger pangs, and before I knew it, I would be once again on the drive-through queue. In retrospect, I now more fulsomely appreciate the conditioning of our unconscious mind by the repetitive bombardment of advertisements from fast food chains. It is as though, without realizing it, we become conditioned rats on the treadmill, where intelligent rational thought is flushed away in response to our unconscious drive. The message is "take off the rose-coloured glasses", and develop a sense of mental discipline. In relation to this, ask yourself, "Am I really hungry or is this just an ongoing habit because I am bored or depressed?"

I am sure we have all been guilty of this at various points in our lives when under stress, and certainly my professional responsibilities seemed highly stressful. As a result, after work and on the weekends, I would tend to watch television and became the ultimate couch potato. During commercial breaks, I would almost as if in a hypnotic trance wander by the fridge to make ham sandwiches and eat whatever was available, whether potato chips, leftovers from the night before or chocolate. In this context, my body mass progressively increased, and to my disgust I was now weighing in at 104 kilograms.

Enter my saviour, Michael Hogg. Much of my work involves interstate consulting, and in this regard I regularly attend Sydney to see clients and provide evidence to Courts of Law. This compounded the problem as frequently after work, particularly in the setting of having no immediate family to curtail my activities, instead of being drawn to the fridge, I would attend various restaurants close to my apartment. I am very fortunate to live in a harbour-side apartment in Sydney with some of the finest eateries within 100 metres of the front door. On one occasion, when a very close friend was visiting from overseas for an extended stay, we would retire to Jimmy Liks restaurant for a meal and several martinis at the end of each day. It was during one such dinner sojourn that I was introduced to Michael Hogg by a friend. I was immediately impressed with Michael's energy and zest for life as well as his appearance, which suggested that he was much younger than his stated age. He started speaking with great enthusiasm about the age-nostic lifestyle, stating that even burnt-out tubby professionals such as myself could have a second crack at the title with self-discipline, medical guidance and the motivation to do so.

Ours was a long courtship. When Michael eventually invited me to contribute my expertise to this book, he introduced me to one of its co-authors, Dr. Michael Zachariah. The two of them expounded the virtues of losing weight, and in this context I resolved that I would have a last role of the die and attempt a medically supervised low calorie diet. I was highly sceptical, but nonetheless determined to push forward with the idea, particularly as it was to be medically supervised.

For the past 14 years, my weight has yo-yoed more frequently than a bungee jumper leaping from the Brooklyn Bridge. It is a constant struggle for men on the wrong side of 40 to maintain a regimen of exercise, healthy eating and body mindfulness. Inevitably, as a consequence, it is easy to develop a habit of comfort eating in order to ward off relentless pressures to perform professionally, maintain a family and deal with the inner struggle of recognizing one's encroaching mortality. With the effluxion of time, the continuous bombardment of long lunches, dinners, comfort eating and alcohol takes its toll. Beyond the spread of our waistline, it is harder to recover from a heavy night as we get older and typically we awaken feeling groggy, guilty and in more despair as to the helplessness we feel in terms of curtailing this process.

Prior to commencing my age-nostic diet, I had spoken with one of my daughters, Gabby, a woman with an intimidating intellect. We were discussing what constitutes masculinity. To this she responded, "Real men look after themselves". This aphorism, simple as it is, completely hit the nail on the head for me. I recognized that for many years I had neglected looking after myself in the context of ongoing depression and a nagging feeling that the better part of my life had already been spent. It is interesting that women, young and old, tend to relate to men according to how men relate to themselves. As my discussion with Gabby unfolded, it dawned on me that it is very unsexy, uncool and off-putting to women to encounter a man who does not hold himself in sufficient regard to look after his health. This was the motivational cue I needed to commence the rebirth of my body shape.

Shortly afterwards, a large box arrived at my apartment containing vitamin and mineral supplements for the next six weeks, a booklet and medication to assist in the burning of fat with diet suppressants. I read the extraordinary claim with interest that if I stuck to the diet (500 calories per day), I could lose up to 400 grams per day. "Bullshit" was my initial response, but then I reasoned I had nothing to lose and methodically attended the local butcher's to order specific quantities of meat (100 grams) per portion, as well as a range of healthy vegetables, which I had assiduously avoided for a decade.

The first week was wobbly. My body felt the jolt immediately, although to protect me somewhat I was advised to spend two days before the commencement of the diet eating whatever I liked in order to create additional fat reserves to lessen the blow. Despite this, I persevered, expecting to wake up the following day without my unsightly gut. Needless to say, this did not occur. I was advised to be "patient" and certainly by week two I started to notice subtle changes. These included a clear loss of weight around the face resulting in the gradual disappearance of my double chin, as well as some reduction in my man boobs and girth. People were beginning to comment on my changed appearance. By week three, the process was accelerating. I was now hooked and noticed that in addition to clear signs of body change, my mood and sleep were improving as were my energy levels. I was no longer having the need for a sleep at the end of the working day and I was regaining control of my weekends by requiring less snooze time on Saturday afternoons.

At the time of writing, my goal is to lose 13 kilograms. It should be comparatively easy once I adjust to the low calorie intake and the rude shock this presents to my psyche. The medication, however, assists in reducing my appetite to the point where I am becoming more cognizant that much of my eating, in fact, was habitual rather than spurred by pure need. Boring as this may seem, the positive reinforcement I enjoyed through watching the kilos fall off on a near daily basis (if you stick to the diet, you do in fact lose between 400 and 500 grams per day) more than compensates for the abandonment of this destructive habit. I also noticed that my self-esteem began to improve and that I enjoyed shopping.

I can consequently say that I am a work in progress and that at any age, a healthier diet and lifestyle indeed works. All that is required is the motivation and insight to take the first step, which like any long journey is extremely hard.

The beauty of this diet is that it is rapid and in the process, as I understand it, one's brain chemistry is re-jigged so that the prior level of appetite is replaced with a far more realistic and healthy one. My attitude to food has changed and I am optimistic that I will be able to maintain my new baseline weight. In order to do this, I have finally accepted that some foods are simply off-limits, probably for life, particularly those with high carbohydrate content. This includes chips and things from fast food outlets such as McDonald's. I have now mentally wiped these from my food list. I have also commenced reading widely on the topic in terms of healthy versus non-healthy foods. One book I found particularly helpful is Wheat Belly *by Dr. William Davis, a leading US cardiologist, which provides a scathing appraisal of wheat in the 21st century, claiming that it does not even remotely resemble the type of wheat eaten in primordial times.*

I am still somewhat in grief at having to part company with fast food, although arising from the substantial progress I have made, I now firmly believe with a high degree of confidence that I will be able to avoid this type of eating from now into the future. The fat that I am burning is being gradually replaced by muscle, which metabolizes far more quickly. Who knows, I may consider attempting to run in the Veteran Olympics in 2016.

An Age-nostic Diet

So what do you eat when you want to roll back the years and really start reversing the ageing process? There is rarely anything startlingly revolutionary in the world of dieting and nutrition because there is so little new that has come to light. It is true that seemingly everyday new diets appear like tulips popping up each spring. Good examples of this include the Pritikin diet, the low carb diet, the low fat diet, the high protein diet, the Mediterranean diet, the Hollywood diet...the list literally goes on and on. If these diets are so good, why are new ones constantly being thought up? It could be that it is very good business, having grown into a billion-dollar industry. It is likely to continue growing as we become more obese and continue to eat the wrong things, especially as we get older.

The human body has been evolving for thousands of years and we need to ask ourselves whether what most people eat today is what they are supposed to consume. Given the proportion of overweight and obese people, it would seem our evolution hasn't kept pace with what hits our meal tables. Perhaps it never will, and we will see death rates rise considerably over the next 20 years as we try to cope with this situation.

When we are under constant stress, we eat too much and often choose the easiest and most convenient solution instead of something healthy, which can take valuable time to find or prepare. We also consume more alcohol as a form of relief, even though this only makes us more stressed in the longer term. I am sure anyone that has had a big night out and drank too much knows the feeling, and it only gets much worse as we get older. A few drinks, especially red wine, is a good way to relax; but for most of us it takes a lot of discipline to just stop at two glasses when we are under stress. I would be the first to put my hand up and say I have failed many times when under stress to stop at a reasonable level.

The same goes for sugary foods. Sugar is the worst poison invented by man and the most potent ageing product I know. If sugar was discovered today, it would probably be illegal, but it is now so ingrained in our society that we all take it for granted. A simple look at the number of people who suffer from diabetes is an indication of how attractive sugar is for us all. Many experts now believe that the over-dispensing of sugar to our children is a major factor in them developing addictions later in life, especially alcohol.

Carbohydrates – often called "comfort food" – are another food that we consume in large quantities when we are stressed. There are many other dietary problems that we could discuss and scare the living daylights out of the average man, but that is not what I want to do.

An Age-nostic Approach to Dieting

I can't say the age-nostic diet is entirely revolutionary, but it does seem to work. In the first instance, if you are overweight or just plain obese, there are two key diet programmes that work and you should seriously consider.

If you need any proof, re-read Tim Watson-Munro's piece which outlines his experience with this diet, combined with a treatment of peptides. Even if you are not in too bad a shape but want to feel better, these simple basic rules will help you. If you can stick to this approach, you will keep the weight off and feel healthier.

- Anything white is basically not good and you should restrict intake whenever possible. Such items include bread and white rice (except basmati).
- Avoid cereals of most kinds (they are all full of sugar).
- Avoid any sugar, including sweets, chocolate bars and many so-called health bars which are simply sweets in sheepskin clothing.
- Avoid alcohol – for many of us, most calories in our modern lives are taken in the form of alcohol. If you can't give it up completely (which is true for most of us), try and stick to the following:
  two or three alcohol days per week
  the best drink for weight management is vodka, soda and fresh lime
  stay away from beer
  if you must drink wine, drink red wine.
- Avoid fruit in the morning before 10am as it is full of sugar and turns straight into calories.
- No chips! Or only once a week at most.
- Stay away from butter, cream and milk products.
- Drink black coffee, not white (but tea is better).
- Only have fried food once a week.
- Only have dessert once a week.
- Don't put any sauce on your food and use only healthy dressings like olive oil and balsamic vinegar.

Cutting the calorie intake is half the battle. The other part is upping the burn. You have to exercise but forget the personal trainer. You will end up hating him or falling in love with her. Walk, walk, walk! That will make such a difference. Walk for at least an hour each day as fast as you can without jogging, as if you are late for a job interview or first date.

As you can see, the age-nostic diet is quite straightforward. Nearly all of the diets that have ever been designed are simply unsustainable and really quite useless. The statistics of people, both men and women, who don't stick to such diet programmes are scary. I really believe if you can stick to these simple rules outlined here, you can lose a lot of weight and will feel as though you will be able to stay on this programme for an extended period. Moreover, you won't feel deprived of the basic enjoyment of eating which can be one of life's greatest pleasures. I love my food with a passion but I do try and stick to the rules I have set out here.

As I put pen to paper today at the tender age of 53 years, I am just under 80 kilos in weight. This is the same weight as I was on my 21st birthday although I am much fitter now than then. I love exercise, but with all my travelling there is no way that I can do it every day. If I miss a day or even two, I will make this up by working out harder and for longer. The many supplements I take are not for losing weight; they are for maintaining a healthy body.

Many men fail to realize that a lot of the weight they carry is just plain water or fluid retention and many foods that we eat make this condition much worse. Have you ever noticed after a big night on the drink that you look bloated in the mirror? This is due to fluid retention, and if you keep up the heavy drinking, you will develop a wonderful pudgy face. Look at any heavy drinker and his face will always be quite pudgy, not to mention the famous double chin that has almost become commonplace these days on business executives.

A tip: if you are going to have a big night out or a busy week of socializing, then drink lots of water before, during and after plus take some fluid retention supplements bought from a health food store. Get the natural ones that are very good and safe. It is also worth remembering that alcohol is a depressant. You should always take some magnesium and 5http before you go out and the day after to help with the post night-out blues. If you drink regularly, take these supplements daily. But generally try to give up the big nights.

In summary, I wish I could give you a wonderful new revolutionary diet plan for the man over 40 years of age that would transform your body in the quickest time possible. But I truly believe there isn't one, and even if there was, you wouldn't stick to it anyway. My advice is to be pragmatic and do the best you can. Stick to the recommendations above and you will get back in shape and, as you see results, this will lead to more enthusiasm. Alcohol is one of the biggest contributory factors in weight gain for men, especially for those over 40 years old, so make sure you focus your efforts of improvement on this tricky area.

Preventing the Big C

Most cancers appear later in life. In particular, the statistics for prostate cancer in men are alarming. It is the biggest killer, but it is also one of the most preventable cancers. We see the signs early in a number of areas but, men being men, we tend to ignore them and plough on regardless, hoping that everything will be OK. Usually, things are OK, but as we get older, we do have to start taking these signs seriously.

As far as prostate cancer is concerned, the best thing you can do is get tested. Have your PSA checked by blood test. Go one step further by seeing your doctor and getting him to check your prostate digitally. This does not mean via the Internet or cable TV, but a simple examination whereby your doctor basically puts his finger into your rear and manually checks your prostate. Not pleasant unless you like that sort of thing, but much quicker than getting a tooth filled or collecting a parking ticket off your car windscreen – and it could save your life.

I strongly believe in antioxidant food and its power to prevent cancers. Much research suggests they protect you from many forms of cancer if only you can somehow include them into your regular diet. They will protect you against free radicals which many experts believe are a big cause of cancer. Sorry to tell you but there are no hamburgers, chips, ice cream, sausages or any other comfort foods on that list. Still, here it is – try hard to get them into your diet, and as much as possible, especially if you are aged 40-plus.

Top 10 Antioxidant Foods

Berries—*blueberries, raspberries and blackberries contain proanthocyanidins, which are antioxidants and may help in preventing cancer as well as heart disease.*

Broccoli—*along with other vegetables such as cabbage, cauliflower and Brussels sprouts, broccoli may help in preventing cancer and heart disease.*

Tomatoes—*lycopene is the key ingredient in the highly versatile tomato. Lycopene is also found in pink grapefruit and, according to recent research, men who eat more tomatoes benefit from lower rates of prostate cancer.*

Red grapes—*these contain reservatrol and quercetin which are potent antioxidants and keep blood vessels open. Reservatrol is believed to assist in the prevention of cancer, gastric ulcers, strokes and potentially osteoporosis.*

Garlic—*it has been shown to help prevent heart disease and cancer as well as slow down the ageing process. It is also an excellent anti-fungal.*

Spinach—*this helps protect our vision because it contains lutein. Studies show spinach-eaters are less likely to develop cataracts or macular degeneration.*

Green tea—*this can significantly reduce the risk of stroke, heart disease and cancer. As well as making a refreshing brew, it can also be added to foods.*

Carrots—*these are full of beta-carotene, which helps in the fight against cancer and can stop arthritis from progressing. Cooking breaks down active compounds within carrots, making them more available.*

Whole grains—*these contain vitamin E, which is a strong antioxidant that can help prevent prostate cancer. It also helps reduce the risks of breast, liver and colon cancers.*

Prunes—*these actually have the highest antioxidant value as measured by the Oxygen Radical Absorbance Capacity. Not a lot of people know that!*

FORMER FAT BAST**D

Ten tips for age-nostic drinking:
1. If you really want to drink, then stick to vodka.
2. Don't drink during the day.
3. It's alright to have a blowout occasionally.
4. A hangover will make you depressed.
5. Take vitamin pills if you are going on a big night.
6. Don't drink when you fly.
7. Don't drink beer unless you want to get fat.
8. Don't drink too much wine as the sulphide content will make you feel lousy.
9. We already know when we have a problem – it's a question of doing something about it.
10. Limit drinking to two to three days per week.

Ten tips for age-nostic eating:
1. You can't eat as if you are still 20 years old.
2. Avoid anything white if you want to lose weight.
3. One blowout a week is OK.
4. Watch your red meat consumption as our ability to digest it falls markedly as we get older.
5. If you are not exercising, limit your calorie intake.
6. Eat anti-ageing and cancer-preventing foods.
7. Don't go past the tipping point with your weight.
8. You can lose all those kilos if you really want to.
9. Drink two litres of water per day.
10. Don't eat junk food.

Ten Great Anti-ageing Foods:

Avocado—this is one of the most alkalizing foods available. Avocados are very high in vitamin E which is essential for glowing skin and shining hair. It also helps keep those wrinkles off your face. Have a raw avocado salad or a steamed one with some salt to add effect.

Berries—*all berries, especially gooseberries, are very rich in vitamin C and therefore highly useful to the body. Vitamin C helps in proper blood circulation and provides minerals and salts to all the body parts. Needless to say, this helps the body to fight against ageing and keep fit.*

Green vegetables—*broccoli, spinach, lettuce, salad leaves and other such greens are highly beneficial for the body. Not only do they help keep the body weight low, they also help fight toxins. Fighting toxins is important because a highly toxic body is like a magnet for all kinds of diseases that can harm the body.*

Garlic—*this is one of the most important foods provided to us by nature. The benefits of garlic are numerous. It helps prevent cell degeneration, helps keep the blood thin and also prevents heart diseases. It is most beneficial when eaten raw.*

Ginger—*this root facilitates digestion and is therefore essential for the body. Ginger keeps bowel movement in shape, thereby enabling good gut health.*

Nuts—*almonds and cashew nuts are like powerhouses of energy. Consuming nuts on a daily basis will fight that lethargic feeling and fill the body with immense energy.*

Yogurt—*rich in important minerals like potassium, calcium, protein and B vitamins. Apart from these, what makes yogurt one of the most powerful foods is the presence of live bacteria in it. This bacteria helps absorption of nutrients in the intestines and stabilizes the immune system.*

Whole wheat pasta and brown rice—*carbohydrates are long-term energy foods and should never be given up unless you want to invite trouble. Substitute white pasta and rice with whole wheat pasta and brown rice and you will instantly feel the difference in your energy level.*

Melons—*water melons and musk melons not only have an alkalizing effect on the body, they also provide the body with essential fluids that it needs for performing various tasks.*

Water—*nothing compares to water. Stay away from those aerated drinks for it takes 32 glasses of water to balance out the ill effects of one glass of soda. Water is essential for our body. It flushes out all the toxins from the body. It also provides fluidity for the flow of blood. At least eight glasses of clean pure water must be consumed on a daily basis.*

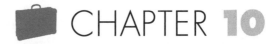

CHAPTER **10**

DON'T MAKE ME RUN!

Getting and staying in age-nostic shape

I have always tried to keep fit and it is the one discipline that I have not failed at. Fitness is the backbone of so many things. Feeling great and beating depression have been two of the most obvious for me. Exercise lifts dopamine levels and this is why we always feel so good after doing it. It probably also has a lot to do why we always felt great when we were children.

When I was a child, we all just raced around, doing amazing amounts of exercise without even knowing it. The fat boy was so rare at school – like one or two in a class of 30 – he was the one ridiculed and bullied the most because he was different. Today, this has completely reversed and it is the skinny nerd who is bullied by all the fat boys. Imagine today if every man over 40 with a huge belly and double chin was ridiculed because of the way he looked. It would be chaos. But sadly there would be too few others to ridicule them because basically we are all in the same boat.

What amazes me is the acceptance of obesity in men, especially those over 40; it seems society now accepts this as the norm today. Physical attractiveness should never be the most important thing in any man, of course, but why is obesity so accepted and mitigated by money and success?

I recently went to an anti-ageing conference in Las Vegas and decided to visit the casino in the hotel where we were staying. What a shock that was! It wasn't the hundreds of people mindlessly sitting in front of machines getting their exercise from pulling down a rather light handle; it was that I had clearly missed out on one of the greatest business opportunities of my life.

I should have invented or sold electric wheelchairs! I was astounded to see the number of men driving around in them – any dodgem car race I had enjoyed as a child failed in comparison to this scene. They were neither old nor infirm – they were mostly in their 50s – but there were so many of them and all obese. What was also incredible was that they did not look particularly unhappy or self-conscious. In fact, most had a drink in hand, a big smile on their face and the intent and focus of a hunting dog heading as quickly as they could to wherever they were heading. I said to Dr. Zacharia, who was with me at the conference, "Look at this! How did this happen?" In the meantime, in the room above, there were some 2,000 doctors talking about reversing and slowing the ageing process.

It's not just at casinos where this new breed of man hangs out. Go to any American airport and have a good look around and prepare to be astounded. Recently I was waiting for a flight in the US and started counting the obese men against what I considered a healthy-looking man. I finally found one of the latter when I boarded the plane – he was the flight attendant collecting our tickets! In the US, the staff on planes are older, and he was clearly in his late 40s. I guessed he was gay and that he had to stay in shape to attract a partner.

I have gay friends almost all over 40, and I have always been fascinated why gay men keep themselves in so much better shape than heterosexual men at that age. You rarely see an obese gay man; the majority are in great shape. My own conclusion for this is that they are not in a traditional relationship, most are single, or simply the older man is trying to attract a younger partner and needs to compete and look his best.

The health benefits for these men as they get older are obvious, so it makes me wonder why the average heterosexual man over 40 – married or single –seems to be the opposite of their gay counterpart. Maybe my "fat buddy" theory really does have something to do with it: "If every other guy looks this way, why shouldn't I?"

When my editor suggested I include a chapter on exercise, I looked at him like a dog being shown a card trick. There are already hundreds of books on the subject, one of the most recent being the hugely successful *4-Hour Body* (by Timothy Ferris). And although I exercise regularly, I am no expert. At that time, I was staying at Home House in London and using the gym each day. While doing so, I noticed an incredibly fit man teaching a Pilates class, and afterwards we immediately struck up a conversation. Now this guy is really fit which, let's face it, a personal trainer should be. Jonathon has huge energy and the most important quality in any man, a great sense of humour, and we quickly started to banter. Furthermore, Jonathon is 47 years old. After only two sessions of Pilates, I took the plunge and said, "Jonathon, you don't really know me, but life is full of opportunities. Could we have a coffee so I could talk to you about an opportunity?" He must have thought I was going to ask him to take a package to Australia for me from my accent!

I told him I was writing a book about anti-ageing for men and asked whether he would be interested in contributing to the chapter on exercise. He trusted me but I think he was just relieved that I was not a drug runner. I thanked him for his trust and we have now become good friends. He has also got me even fitter.

Before we get on to Jonathon's story and his exercise programme for the age-nostic man, it's worth stressing that running on treadmills and doing weights alone is not going to get you into shape. In parallel to exercise, you need to consider everything covered in the previous chapter on diet and food. Read that chapter again and then start some exercise, and keep to it until the day you can no longer do so. Common sense rears its ugly head again!

Always remember the "old devil on the shoulder" joke. On the left shoulder, he is whispering into your ear:

"Go sit and watch TV, have some fast food and have a beer. You're too tired for that rubbish. It won't do you much good anyway. Go on, give up, you know you want to."

And on the right shoulder, he is saying:

"Just do it! You will feel great. You are looking so much better. She's finding you more attractive; your friends are commenting on how great you are looking. You can even now see your penis when you look down! You are looking younger and your mood is fantastic!"

TURN RIGHT AS MUCH AS YOU CAN.

The Age-nostic Exercise Regime
By Jonathan Goodair

I can still remember when I was a kid, looking at the older people around me and thinking, "How did they come to look like that?" Hunched shoulders, fat belly, saggy faces, moving awkwardly, huffing and puffing at the least exertion. It seemed to me that the older people got, the less like human beings they actually looked. I knew from this time that I did not want this to happen to me and I had to do everything I could to prevent it.

Age is inevitable; we are all going to get older and deteriorate, but it's how we age that is important.

During the early part of my career, I worked as an instructor and personal fitness trainer in various gyms in central London. Eventually, I was invited to become one of the personal trainers working under the supervision of Australian Strength and Conditioning specialist, David Crottie. I spent seven years with David in his business, and during this time, I realized that there was something missing from what we did – all that running, jumping, weight lifting, sit-ups and eating did pay off, but you ended up all puffed up and big and not very flexible. I felt that training needed more refining, the ideal programme and the ideal body somewhere between a bodybuilder and a ballet dancer.

I started to learn about Pilates as ballet dancers use this to strengthen their bodies in a way that doesn't bulk out the muscles. It improves coordination and flexibility, or rather it doesn't improve flexibility but you need good flexibility to get the best from doing it. Pilates is exercise performed in good posture, developing a body that is able to maintain good posture when the body is under strain. It makes you walk taller or rather it makes it much easier for you to walk tall, sit upright and move your body in the way it was designed to move. As we get older, our posture starts to deteriorate for a number of reasons, including developing bad postural habits. Pilates will help you to reverse this process.

Lifting heavy weights, running distances, sitting at a desk for long periods and being tired all encourage poor posture and alignment. So if you exercise, challenge the body in good alignment, then the body will become stronger in a more functional way and you will find it easier to maintain perfect posture with much less physical and mental effort. The danger with Pilates and yoga is that most people do not have the flexibility/mobility in their bodies to perform these exercises correctly; their spines do not articulate in the correct areas so all the movement (articulation) takes place at the wrong point.

These people need one-to-one guidance as to which exercises to perform and which to avoid. Their exercises need to be adjusted to accommodate their various ailments or restrictions. They need to be prescribed exercises that will allow them to move correctly. Specific muscles need to be targeted for stretching/lengthening. Exercises need to be filtered so that you don't waste time on exercises that either are not suitable to your body type/shape or that don't contribute to the end goal. I believe that by combining specific Pilates, strength and conditioning exercises you can develop a long, lean, muscular body that is pain-free and moves with ease.

After my years under David Crottie's umbrella, I moved to Home House (HH), a private members' club in London's Portman Square, which is a much smaller gym but under my control. Here I further refined my mixture of Pilates, strength and conditioning. I eventually came to the attention of Madonna as she was training with a guy who had also trained me, James D'Silva. James was a former ballet dancer and choreographer who had set up his own Pilates studio and he was Madonna's trainer, which in my book was quite something. I was asked to take Madonna through a trial Pilates routine at HH. After the workout, she said, "Now I know that you're a real trainer I'll be back", and she was true to her word.

James was very helpful to me. I would go to his studio daily with Madonna and watch and learn from the master. When James wasn't available I would step in; it was a fantastic experience. I applied what I was doing with James and Madonna to my routines and the results were fantastic. After a couple of years, Madonna introduced me to another well-known celeb. This was the start of working with some very high-profile people. Again I learned a lot and applied this to what I already knew. I specialized in women's training for the next couple of years featuring in Vogue, Elle, The Times, The Daily Telegraph, Stella Magazine, Hello and many more.

Participation Readiness
Most people should check with their doctor before beginning an exercise programme. Before embarking on your training regime, answer the questions

below. If you are over 69 years of age and you are not physically active, you should certainly check with your doctor before beginning any exercise programme. If you are aged between 50 and 69, answering the questions below will tell you if you need to see a doctor before beginning.

1. *Has your doctor ever told you that you have a heart condition AND that you should only do physical activity recommended by a doctor?*

2. *Do you feel pain in your chest when you do physical activity?*

3. *In the past months, have you had chest pain when you were not doing physical activity?*

4. *Do you lose your balance because of dizziness or do you ever lose consciousness?*

5. *Do you have a bone or joint problem that could be made worse by a change in your physical activity?*

6. *Is your doctor currently prescribing drugs for your blood pressure or heart condition?*

7. *Do you know of any other reason why you should not do physical activity?*

If you answer yes to one or more of these questions, talk with your doctor before you start becoming more physically active. If you answered no to all of the questions, you can be reasonably sure you can start to become much more active. Start slowly and build up gradually.

Exercise Recommendations

It is worth studying the pictures closely to get familiar with exactly how your body should move during these key exercises. It is worth doing many of these in front of a mirror to ensure correct posture and positioning. I can't stress this enough, as some exercises can do harm if not performed properly.

In an ideal standing posture you should be able to draw a plumb line that goes straight down through the ear, shoulder, hip, knee and ankle. By strengthening your body in this ideal posture, you are making it easier for your body to maintain this posture. By putting your body under stress in a good posture, you are making it easier for your body to maintain good posture when not under stress. It is important to have a daily routine of stretching in order to maintain good posture and pain-free movement. Ideally make this part of your morning routine.

Aim to perform cardiovascular exercise three to five days every week for 20 to 60 minutes if the intensity is high and a minimum of 30 to 60 minutes if the intensity is low.

Aim to perform resistance exercise two to five days per week.

Aim to perform the stretches every day.

It is important to build up your workout schedule gradually. Begin by only using cardiovascular workouts 1 and 3 for a few weeks to build up some fitness before attempting the higher intensity workout 2.

Sample Weekly Schedule for Beginner Exerciser

Day 1—Warm-up, cat stretch, side bend, spinal rotation, shell stretch, front of thigh stretch, lying hamstring stretch, glute stretch, chest stretch.

Day 2—Warm-up, cat stretch, side bend, spinal rotation, shell stretch, front of thigh stretch, lying hamstring stretch, glute stretch, chest stretch. Cardio routine number 3. Stretches.

Day 3—Warm-up, cat stretch, side bend, spinal rotation, shell stretch, front of thigh stretch, lying hamstring stretch, glute stretch, chest stretch. Core workout, upper body workout. Stretches.

Day 4—Warm-up, cat stretch, side bend, spinal rotation, shell stretch, front of thigh stretch, lying hamstring stretch, glute stretch, chest stretch. Cardio routine number 1, lower body workout. Stretches.

Day 5—Warm-up, cat stretch, side bend, spinal rotation, shell stretch, front of thigh stretch, lying hamstring stretch, glute stretch, chest stretch. Cardio routine number 3, core workout, upper body workout. Stretches.

Day 6—Stretches.

Day 7—Stretches.

Sample Weekly Schedule for Current Exerciser

Day 1—Warm-up, cat stretch, side bend, spinal rotation, shell stretch, front of thigh stretch, lying hamstring stretch, glute stretch, chest stretch. Cardio routine number 1, core workout, upper body workout. Stretches.

Day 2—Warm-up, cat stretch, side bend, spinal rotation, shell stretch, front of thigh stretch, lying hamstring stretch, glute stretch, chest stretch. Cardio routine number 2, core workout, lower body workout. Stretches.

Day 3—Warm-up, cat stretch, side bend, spinal rotation, shell stretch, front of thigh stretch, lying hamstring stretch, glute stretch, chest stretch. Cardio routine number 3. Stretches.

Day 4—Warm-up, cat stretch, side bend, spinal rotation, shell stretch, front of thigh stretch, lying hamstring stretch, glute stretch, chest stretch. Cardio routine number 1, core workout, upper body workout. Stretches.

Day 5—Warm-up, cat stretch, side bend, spinal rotation, shell stretch, front of thigh stretch, lying hamstring stretch, glute stretch, chest stretch. Cardio routine number 2, core workout, lower body workout. Stretches.

Warm-up and Stretch

Before working out, it's important to go through a series of stretches to lengthen the muscles and prepare the body for exercise.

WARM-UP upper body

Stand with your feet hip distance apart, shoulders relaxed. Lengthen up through the crown off your head, tuck your tail bone slightly and draw in your belly button.

SHOULDER ROLLS forward then back × 5–10

Roll your shoulders back in large circles then forward. Draw your arms back to open your chest, lift up your heart and keep your collar bones wide.

HEAD TURNS left and right × 3 each way

Reaching up through the crown of your head, turn your head to look over your right shoulder then left shoulder.

ARM CIRCLES forward/back × 5–10

Relax your shoulders and make large circles with your arms, back then forward. Draw your arms back to open your chest, lift up your heart and keep your collar bones wide.

SIDE STRETCHES × 3 each side

Widen your stance to shoulder distance apart. Stretch your right arm up and over to the side, reaching through your fingertips. Keep your hips still.

CAT STRETCHES × 4-8

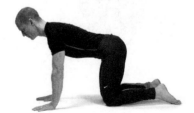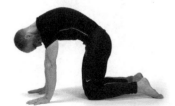

On hands and knees, hands are shoulder distance apart, knees are hip distance apart, shoulders over hands and hips over knees. Lengthen through your spine and lift up through the crown of your head. Breathe in to prepare and as you breathe out draw your belly button in, arch your spine up and push your hands into the floor, breathe in as you return to the start position reaching your chest forward and lifting up the tops of your ears.

SIDE BEND x 3 each side

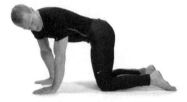
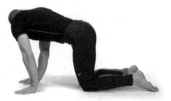

Keep your spine long as you turn to the left and then the right. Look as far round as you can without moving your hips. Focus on the movement in the middle of your spine.

SPINAL ROTATION x 3 each side

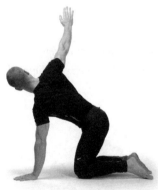
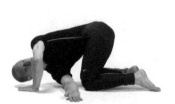

Breathe in as you press down into the floor with your left hand and reach your right arm out to the side and up to the ceiling, follow your hand with your eyes as you reach up through the fingertips. Breathe out as you sweep the arm down and under the body, bending the supporting elbow and reaching through along the floor as far as possible. Try to work through as big a range of motion as possible while maintaining stable hips and torso.

SHELL STRETCH x 5 full relaxed breathes

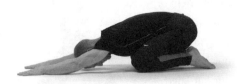

On hands and knees, sit back on to your heels reaching your arms forward along the floor in front of you. Breathe in to the back of the ribs and relax your tailbone down to the floor.

WARM-UP *lower body*

HALF SQUAT x 20

With your arms reaching forward and your feet shoulder-width apart, breathe in and begin to bend your knees. Sit back on your heels, keeping your back straight and eyes forward. Never let your knees go past your toes. Once your legs are bent to near 90 degrees (but not beyond), you can ascend back to the starting position, breathing out as you do. Engage abs all the way down and up.

STRETCHES lower body

KNEELING FRONT OF HIP AND THIGH STRETCH x 30–90 seconds

To stretch the left FRONT of HIP and THIGH muscles, take a kneeling lunge position, right knee on the floor, bring your left foot far enough forward to feel a stretch on the front of your right hip. With your right arm by your side, breathe out as you reach the right arm forward and up, gently moving your hips forward, tucking your tailbone slightly and lifting your chest to increase the stretch. Your left knee should be over your left ankle.

KNEELING HAMSTRING STRETCH x 30–90 seconds

Now move your hips backwards to stretch the muscles on the BACK of the LEFT THIGH. Lengthen your spine, flex your left foot and push out behind you with your left hip to lengthen your hamstrings.

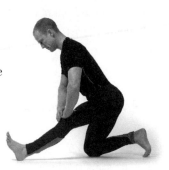

OR

LYING HAMSTRING STRETCH x 30–90 seconds

Lie on your back with your knees bent and feet flat on the floor. Using a yoga strap or towel to hook over your right foot, slowly pull the strap to straighten your right leg as much as possible while pressing the back of your right hip into the floor to deepen the stretch. Now slide your left leg out on the floor to further increase the stretch.

GLUTE STRETCH x 30–90 seconds

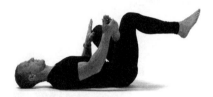

Lying on your back with knees bent and feet flat on the floor, cross your left ankle over your right knee and draw your right knee towards your chest. Press down through the back of your left hip to intensify the stretch.

STRETCHES upper body

CHEST STRETCH
x 30–90 seconds
Standing with feet hip distance apart, clasp your hand together in the small of your back, draw your elbows and shoulders back and lift your chest.

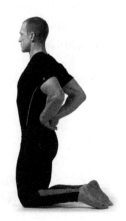

Core (Abdominal) Training 3–5 Days Per Week

CLASSIC ABDOMINAL CRUNCH × 10–20

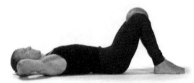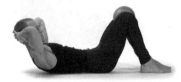

Lie on your back, knees bent and feet flat on the floor. Hands are behind your head, elbows just in your peripheral vision. Breathe in to prepare and as you breathe out draw your belly button in towards your spine, press your lower back into the floor and leading with your ribcage, curl forward, allowing your head to sink into your hands, eyes looking into your belly button. Don't jam your chin down on to your chest; imagine you're trying to hold a ripe peach under your chin. Try to widen your back as you curl forward and keep the width across your collar bones. Breathe in as you return to the start position.

LONG ABDOMINAL CRUNCH × 10–20

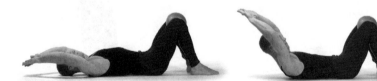

Lying on your back, knees bent and feet flat on the floor. Arms are held straight behind you in line with your ears. Breathe in to prepare and as you breathe out draw your belly button in towards your spine, press your lower back into the floor and leading with your ribcage, curl forward, eyes looking into your belly button. Try to widen your back as you curl forward and keep the width across your collar bones. Breathe in as you return to the start position.

DOUBLE CRUNCH x 10–20

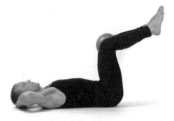 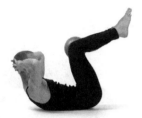

Lie on your back, knees bent and feet flat on the floor. Hands are behind your head, elbows just in your peripheral vision. Breathe in to prepare and as you breathe out draw your belly button in towards your spine, press your lower back into the floor and leading with your ribcage, curl forward, allowing your head to sink into your hands, simultaneously lift your feet off the floor and bring your knees back to meet your elbows. Keep your lower back pressed into the floor throughout. Try to widen your back as you curl forward and keep the width across your collar bones. Breathe in as you return to the start position.

SINGLE OBLIQUE CURL x 10–20

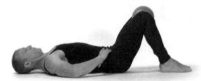 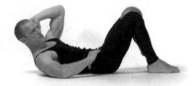

Lie on your back with knees bent and feet flat on the floor. With your left hand behind your head and your right hand on your right hip, breathe in to prepare and as you breathe out, draw your belly button in towards your spine, press your lower back into the floor and leading with your ribcage, curl forward and twist to the right, keeping your left elbow wide. Keep your hips fixed and feel the rotation in the torso. Try to widen your back as you curl forward and keep the width across your collar bones. Breathe in as you return to the start position.

HALF SIDE BRIDGE x 20–40 seconds

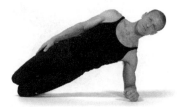

In a side lying position, propped on your left elbow with your left shoulder overhanging your left elbow, line up your shoulder, hip and knee in a straight line. Bend the knees to about 90 degrees. Keeping the alignment between your shoulder, hip and knee, lift your hips up off the floor to form a straight line with your body from your knees to your head. Hold this position, lengthening your body and breathing continuously, feeling the ribcage narrow as you breathe out. Repeat on the right side.

FULL SIDE BRIDGE x 20–60 seconds

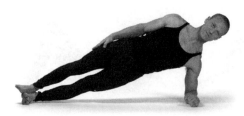

In a side lying position, propped on your left elbow with left shoulder overhanging your left elbow, line up your shoulder, hip and knee and ankle in a straight line. Have one foot on top of the other. Keeping the alignment between your shoulder, hip, knee and ankle, lift your hips up off the floor to form a straight line with your body from your ankles to your head. Hold this position, lengthening your body, breathing continuously and feeling the ribcage narrow as you breathe out.

FULL OBLIQUES × 10–20 pairs

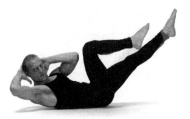 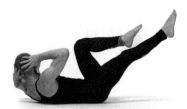

Lie on your back with your feet off the floor and knees above your hips. Hands are behind your head, elbows wide. Breathe in to prepare and as you breathe out, draw your belly button in towards your spine, press your lower back into the floor and leading with your ribcage, curl forward, allowing your head to sink into your hands, eyes looking into your belly button. Don't jam your chin down on to your chest; imagine you're trying to hold a ripe peach under your chin. Try to widen your back as you curl forward and keep the width across your collar bones. Take a short breath in then breathe out, pull in your abs and turn your shoulders to the right and reach your left leg straight forward, keeping your lower back pressed into the floor. Take another short breath in as you return to the start position, then pull in your abs and breathe out, turning to the left side and reaching the right leg forward; take another short breath in as you return to the start position.

REVERSE CRUNCH × 10–20

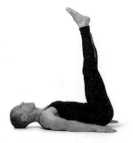 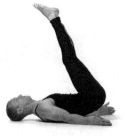

Lie on your back with your feet off the floor and knees at 90 degrees or legs straight up in the air, feet above your hips. Arms are slightly out to the side with palms pressing gently into the floor. Drop your chin down towards your chest slightly. Breathe in to prepare and as you breathe out, press your lower back into the floor and draw your knees towards your chest, allowing the tailbone to curl up off the floor a little, breathe in as you return to the start position pressing your lower back into the floor. On the long leg reverse, don't swing your legs. As you breathe out, pull in your lower abdominals and press down through the back of the ribs and curl your tailbone off the mat, toes travelling towards your forehead. Don't hold your breath.

HALF PLANK x 20–40 seconds

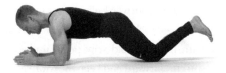

Start on your forearms and knees on the floor, hands clasped together. Position your hips to form a straight line between your knees, hips, shoulders and ears. Tuck your tailbone slightly to engage your lower abdominals. Don't stick your bottom in the air or allow your back to sag down. Breathe continuously and pull in your belly button.

FULL PLANK x 20–40 seconds

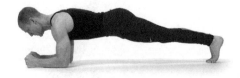

Start on your forearms and knees and feet on the floor, hands clasped together. Lift your knees up off the floor and position your hips to form a straight line between your ankles, knees, hips, shoulders and ears. Tuck your tailbone slightly to engage your lower abdominals. Don't stick your bottom in the air or allow your back to sag down. Breathe continuously and pull in your belly button. If you feel this exercise in your lower back, go back to performing the HALF PLANK.

UPPERBACK EXTENSION × 10–20

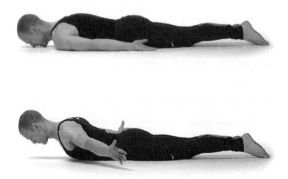

Lie face down on the floor, legs together, arms by your sides with palms facing up. Keep your chin slightly tucked and breathe in to prepare. As you breathe out press your pubic bone into the floor, pull your belly button to your spine and gently draw your shoulders back and down lifting your head and shoulders away from the floor slightly while pressing your lower chest and ribs into the floor. Breathe in as you return to the start position.

Cardiovascular Training 3–5 Days Per Week and 150–300 Minutes Per Week

Energy for low intensity and longer duration exercise comes predominately from stored body fat. Target heart rate 60% of maximum, effort level feels "fairly light".

Energy for moderate intensity exercise comes from a mixture of stored body fat and energy stored in the muscles and liver. Target heart rate 70-80%

of maximum. Effort level feels "somewhat hard".

Energy for high intensity short duration exercise comes predominately from energy stored in the muscles. Target heart rate 90-100% of maximum. Effort level feels very hard.

To calculate your target heart rate, subtract your age from 220 and multiply by the desired percentage. For example, 46-year-old wants to work at 80%, 220-46 = 174. Therefore 174bpm = max heart rate. 174×80% = 174×0.8 = 139. Target heart rate = 139bpm.

Cardio day 1.

- Choose one or a combination of the following: run/walk/bike/cross trainer/swim/row.
- 5-minute warm-up easy pace.
- 15-30 minutes moderate intensity 70-80% effort.
- 5 minutes cool-down easy pace.
- Stretches then run/bike/cross trainer/rowing machine.

Cardio day 2.

- Choose one or a combination of the following: run/walk/bike/cross trainer/swim/row.
- Warm-up 5 minutes easy pace 80-100% effort, light resistance.
- 40 seconds at high intensity (maximum effort), 20 seconds low intensity × 10 rounds.
- Cool-down 5 minutes easy pace.
- Stretches.

Cardio day 3.

- Choose one or a combination of the following: run/walk/bike/cross trainer/swim/row.
- 30-60 minutes low intensity 60-70% effort.
- Stretches.

ALWAYS STRETCH AFTER WORKING OUT.

Lower Body Workout

The CLASSIC BUTT KICK × 10–30 reps

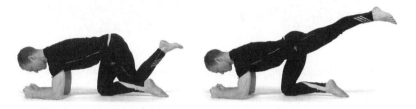

On forearms and knees, arms shoulder distance apart and knees hip distance apart. Eyes looking straight down, abdominals drawn in and spine straight. Breathe in to prepare and as you breathe out, reach your left leg straight behind and up as high as you can without moving your lower back or pelvis. Straighten your leg fully at the knee with no tension in your thigh. It is important here to maintain width across your back; don't allow the work to go into your neck and shoulders. Focus on maintaining alignment between your neck and spine. Breathe in as you return to start position.

CLASSIC SIDE LEG LIFT × 10–30 reps

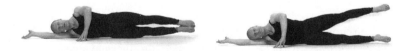

Lying on your side in a long straight line, with your lower arm lengthened along the floor with your ear resting on your bicep. Roll your torso and hips forward a quarter turn in alignment. Breathe in to prepare and as you breathe out, slowly lift the top leg, maintaining length through your whole body. Breathe in as you return to the start position. Shoulders are wide, spine long. Gently draw in your abdominals to stabilize against the movement.

CLASSIC SIDE LYING ADDUCTION × 10–30 reps

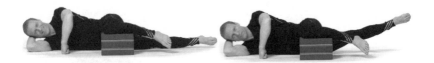

The body should be long and straight as in Classic Side Leg Lift but with your top knee bent to 90 degrees. Breathe in to prepare and as you breathe out, lengthen through your heel and reach through your fingertips as you lift your bottom leg. Keep your torso as still as possible and gently draw in your stomach, breathing in as you lower. When you lift your leg, try not to bend your knee. Keep your shoulders wide and relaxed. There is no movement on any other part of the body other than the leg.

SUPINE HIP EXTENSION × 10–30 reps

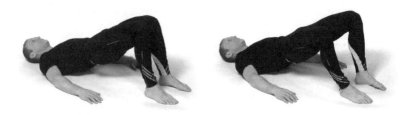

Lie on your back with your arms by your sides, knees bent and feet flat on the floor. Knees and feet are hip distance apart. Breathe in to prepare and as you breathe out, gently press your lower back into the floor, curl your tailbone off the floor and tilt your pelvis up, curling your spine off the floor one vertebra at a time to shoulder blade level. Breathe in and hold the position for one second, then breathe out as you roll your spine and pelvis back on to the floor one vertebra at a time. Focus on keeping your knees hip distance apart.

HALF SQUAT × 10–30 reps

Have your arms reaching forward and shoulders wide and relaxed. Have your feet shoulder-width apart, breathe in and begin to bend your knees. Sit back on your heels, keeping your back straight and eyes forward. Knees are in line with your toes, never letting your knees go past your toes. Once your legs are bent to near 90 degrees (but not beyond), you can ascend back to the starting position, breathing out as you do. Engage abs all the way down and up.

ALWAYS STRETCH AFTER WORKING OUT

Upper Body Workout

For the upper body workout, select a weight that allows you to perform the exercise while maintaining correct posture. If you don't have dumbbells, you can use a book or any other object that is easily held.

SINGLE ARM BICEP CURL WITH OVERHEAD PRESS AND TRICEP EXTENSION COMBO × 10–20 reps

Standing tall, have your feet between hip and shoulder distance apart, knees soft and shoulders wide. Breathe in to prepare and as you breathe

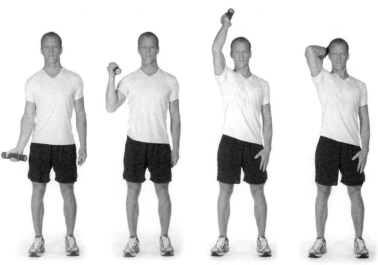

out, pull your belly button in to your spine and bicep curl the dumbbell to your shoulder. Breathe in and straighten your arm up overhead, breathe out as you bend the elbow, lowering the dumbbell behind your head, keeping your upper arm as vertical as possible. Breathe in as you straighten your arm up overhead, breathe out as you lower the dumbbell to your shoulder, and finally breathe in as you return to the start position under control, maintaining an upright posture.

ONE ARM DUMBBELL ROW x 10–20 reps

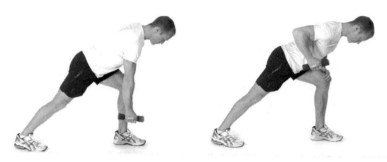

Stand in a long forward lunge position, with your feet hip distance apart and your left hand on your left thigh, supporting your upper body. Your spine should be straight and eyes looking down at the dumbbell in your right hand. Without twisting your torso, begin to slowly bring the dumbbell up to your ribs, exhaling as you do and keeping your elbow as tight as possible into your body. Slowly bring the weight back down to the starting position.

TRICEP KICK BACK x 10–20 reps

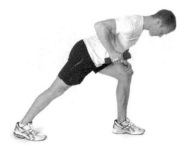 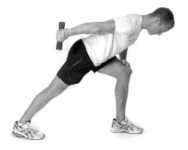

Stand in a long forward lunge position, left foot forward. Your feet should be hip distance apart and your left hand on your left thigh, supporting your upper body. Your spine should be straight and eyes looking down at the dumbbell in your right hand. Start with your right hand held close in to your ribs with your right elbow lifted as much as possible without twisting your torso. Breathe out as you straighten your arm, keeping your right elbow high, belly button pulled into your spine. Breathe in as you return to the start position.

PUSH UP × 10–20 reps

Lie face down on the floor with your hands just wider than your shoulders. Maintaining a straight line through your ankles, knees, hips, shoulders and ears, breathe in to prepare and as you breathe out, pull in your abdominals, tuck in your tailbone slightly and push yourself up until your arms are straight but not locked at the elbow. Breathe in as you return to the start position.

FINALLY, ALWAYS STRETCH AFTER WORKING OUT.

Ten tips for exercising and keeping it up:

1. Identify your perfect role model.
2. Just start a programme – real men are those who look after themselves.
3. And then stay on that programme.
4. Just do it as soon as you are up – don't put it off.
5. Get yourself some great exercise kit.
6. Load up with a great motivational playlist.
7. Notice how good you feel after each exercise workout.
8. Join a gym – it helps you to stay focused.
9. Take a longish hike every day.
10. Remember, you will only get bigger if you don't make a start.

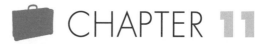

CHAPTER **11**

REDEFINING
RELATIONSHIPS

How our key relationships change over time

Most relationships are good for us. People who enjoy being happily married and have good relationships with a wide circle of friends are more likely to live longer. It is well proven that our mental health has a significant impact on our anti-ageing process. If we are more positive and mentally energetic, we will not only have a more enjoyable life, the chances are we will live longer as well. Good relationships quite simply offer social support, especially in tough times. There is someone to take you to the doctor or to talk to when things become stressful. These kinds of relationships are not built overnight and should be seen as long-term projects. As we get older, many of us place greater emphasis on stable relationships which provide us social support. But when we reach our 40s and 50s, our relationships evolve and change in a way many men are not prepared for.

In our teenage years, friendships and relationships are the most important thing in our lives as we try to assert our personality, create our own stamp and generally spend most of our time building a direction to our life. Our key relationships help shape us, affect what we say, how we act and the very clothes we have on our back. We all had a best friend at school and it was as if life couldn't go forward without that person and their endorsement. Then we quickly discover the opposite sex and before we know it, we have abandoned most of those friendships to pursue a new type of relationship with a new special friend.

As we leave school and start careers, our friends change as everyone goes off on their own path and we create new groups that are usually people we work with or are studying with. These relationships change dramatically as we are trying to get ahead in our careers and we also now have a new father figure in the shape of our boss. He can quickly become our new role model and we are more eager to please him than our paternal father, because he can help us move ahead in our life more than anyone. Quite often this relationship is not a close one and often not really a totally honest one. This is because he is so in charge of our destiny, ambition and financial security that we will do almost anything to show him that we are worthy of a place in his workplace.

Many of our close friendships are also very competitive, as we are competing with our work colleagues for promotions and increased financial rewards. We have also lost many of our former close friends as they have gone off on their own journey. We are in many cases now settling down in a longer-term relationship and this is changing and often quite difficult to deal with. In our 30s, many of our friends are getting married or are in a secure relationship and we lose contact with many of those friends. It can suddenly be a lonely time for men as, slowly but surely, solid friendships slip away. Our male friends are harder to get hold of, we can no longer go out on long nights of partying and we are also getting busier in our careers. Before we know it, the whole dynamic of our friendship circle has changed and we feel a bit disconnected from the secure life we had before.

Another interesting dynamic which I am sure most men can relate to is the situation where we have been in a relationship for some time and then it breaks up. We are suddenly alone, trying to rekindle old friendships again because we want to rebuild those ties, partly to try to generate the same feelings as when we were teenagers.

When we marry and start a family, we become a couple and we start spending time with other couples. Many male friends that are thrust upon us are often the partners of our own partner's friends. We often have little or nothing in common and simply would never choose him as a friend. But as we want to support our partner, we spend endless nights out with this mis-matched friend and in some extreme cases have to even go on holidays with them. This can be a recipe for potential problems as we try and cope with this unison that simply should never have happened.

The next stage of male friendship is after we have had children, when we basically don't seem to have time or energy to have any friends for the first few years. However, this is alleviated by the fact that you have a beautiful new child that is filling up most of your spare time, and you just want to spend as much time as possible with that child and your partner.

Everything has changed so quickly from the simple and solid friendships we had at school, university and work, and before you know it the friendship base has diminished to just a few. Hopefully, you have made the most important decision in your life correctly, which is your choice of partner. I have mentioned before that this is the most important, yet most irrational, decision we seem to make as men. Why else is the divorce rate so high in our 40s and 50s? While we can make incorrect career decisions in our 30s and beyond, we are still able to move on and become more fulfilled. However, one decision we make, often under all the wrong circumstances, can come back to haunt many men as we age. Any relationship can drift and, in many cases, collapse as two people grow differently. Many of us have spent years focusing on our career, moving up the ladder or to new exciting careers, which can lessen the importance of that primary relationship over time. There is certainly no ladder to move up in marriage; we need to live by the choice we made many years ago or run. As I mentioned previously, this can be a major contributory factor towards what a lot of people call the mid-life crisis. By the way, in more cases our partners may have come to the same conclusion, which can make the breakdown of communication worse. However, family commitments and the forward momentum we have built up can keep things together until finally something gives way.

I am definitely the last person on earth to give advice on marriage as I come from a broken family and my own marriage did not last. It is no coincidence that it ended in my late 40s because I had experienced my own mid-life crisis. I have learned something from the whole process, and that is the one rule in life is to make sure you marry your best friend and no one else. Friendships usually last because people have many things in common, connect on so many different levels and have more similar interests. Having children is not enough to bind couples together for the long term as they leave and develop their own lives. Quite simply, this relationship should be the longest and most solid you will ever have. It needs to go through the most challenging times that any friendship can. It will not be like the relationship you have with your children which is forged with so much responsibility and a mixture of conflicting emotions.

The relevance of all of this to the age-nostic lifestyle revolves around timing. The time of life that your marriage or long-term relationship will come under the most pressure is often when other major things are happening. There is no doubt that the years following my own marriage breakdown were the loneliest of my life. You miss literally everything that you had, even the partner that is not speaking to you. In my own divorce, I was so disturbed by how tough my lawyer was at the outset, that I went through the rest of the process without one. I quite liked my wife's lawyer who, while tough, was at least trying to be fair.

Keeping the Relationship Going

I messed up my own marriage and a few relationships since, but in the true age-nostic way, I thought I would at least write as if I was getting advice from someone else, so that I can hopefully get it right myself in the future.

Why do so many relationships break down or indeed end? Like most men, I am performance-based and basically needy. As little boys, we were constantly after attention, especially from our mothers. She was the one who for so many years we relied on, and from an early age, we learned we could not survive without her attention. Something like this carries over into our adult life and spills over into our relationships with all the other women who come into our lives, causing confusion and disappointments.

If you had to put long-term relationships into categories, they would probably look something like this. There are those relationships which operate through distractions and connections such as children, hard-earned assets (home and lifestyle) and the fear of losing any of those things. And when children eventually leave home, or a financial crisis results in the loss of the home or lifestyle, then suddenly the original relationship comes under strain.

Then there are acceptance relationships. While no longer intimate or close, with little or no real communication taking place, the partners get on just enough to stay together without having to break the mold. Habit and security enable life to go on. There are the usual ups and downs, but not enough for either partner to face the future alone.

Then there are the unhappy relationships. The constant tension means life is simply one long battle of attrition. It tires everyone involved until the point of complete breakdown. Partners continue to live under the same roof, but really totally apart. Each takes comfort in any outside distraction or obsession, including affairs, addiction to work or drugs...anything to keep them distracted from having to face or repair the breakdown in their relationship. It continues until both parties reach an age when it is almost pointless and too frightening to contemplate a real break.

And then there is the happy relationship. There is great communication, shared values and interests, mutual respect for each other, a healthy sex life and a general feeling of can't wait to see each other each day. Unfortunately, too many men I know in their 40s-plus do not find themselves in the final category, but in one of the others.

I think the biggest problem with any man, especially as he gets older, is that he tends to forget the simple ways he wooed, or could still woo, any woman he wanted, whether this is to keep or find her. She simply wants you to make her feel as if she is the only person in the room; as if she is the most important person in your life. As we men get older, this seems a real challenge, especially with everything else that is going on with our own mid-life obstacles.

Nevertheless, imagine meeting your partner now for the first time. If you treated her the way you do now, do you think things would last very long between you two? Probably not! The biggest problem in any relationship often centres on attention and intensity which, naturally, over time gets increasingly less. Suddenly she is no longer the most important person in your life; and what you get is exactly what you don't want – less attention and more distance. It's as if you were a young boy again and your mother's care and attention is beginning to wane. It's the greatest catch-22 in life and relationships for men, and I strongly believe men are to blame far more than women.

If I had to give advice to men of 40 and beyond for any relationship, whether it's an existing or new one, then it would be: remember when you were younger. Remember all that attention and energy you focused on your partner; try and still make her feel as if she is the only one in the room, that she is still special, still the one you pursued with such attention and intensity. In an existing relationship, this will help a lot because in actuality she still is all of these things – it's just that you have forgotten over time.

Ultimately, as with everything in this book, it is going to be up to you. As you get older, you need to keep yourself young in body, mind and spirit.

Become as age-nostic in your lifestyle as you can, and she will respond. Turning up at home grumpy and prematurely aged will get you nowhere at all and will only increase the likelihood of the breakdown in your relationship. Even if you have been that "grumpy old man" for a while, by adopting the age-nostic lifestyle and making such efforts to change, in most cases it will light her up because she will respond with the thought that you are doing it for her and the man she fell in love with is on his way back. Well, even if this is stretching it a little, it is the effort that is the important thing, and the most noticeable change will be that you will start talking to her again and showing interest in her life. Energy feeds on energy and communication leads to further communication. Remember those long talks you had about every subject possible when you were first together and how you cared so much about her life, simply because you were in love with her?

If you are looking for a new partner later in life, it goes without saying that getting into good physical shape will be of great help. However, if you still have the energy levels of an old man, then that is exactly how you will be perceived. Your chances of finding happiness again will be reduced and you will either end up alone at home or spending far too much time at work or with other grumpy old men drowning and forgetting themselves in a group setting, further making your health and age decline quicker. There is nothing wrong with becoming a child again!

Breaking Up

Divorce or relationship break-up is an experience not for the fainthearted, but if you do find yourself in a position where things have completely broken down, I will provide a little advice. First, be prepared to suffer some form of depression. You will be thrown completely out of what you knew as life or what you thought was normal. You will be lonelier than you have ever been in your life. Most people I know that have left their partner for someone else have only found that the new relationship that they left the marriage for can break down very quickly.

Every relationship in your life will suffer, especially with your children. You will lose many friends as people choose who to support. Your work will suffer as you are preoccupied with legal matters, change of residence and just the general impact of living on a new planet. It is a horrible and tough time, and it takes a long time to return to any form of happiness. But it does come if you approach it in the right way.

In a lot of cases, you will increase your intake of alcohol because you are feeling totally lost. Just as important is the fact that no one is looking over your shoulder any more. You will go out more because you are looking for new friends and this will cause you to drink more. I am a very social, gregarious person and I found the first months of being alone totally frightening, having to interact as one instead of two. Being on your own can also lead to not eating as well. It can be different and like everything in life, it doesn't need to be this way. Life is not over and you shouldn't think it is, but it takes a huge amount of strength to get through it. If you can remain positive, it can feel like a very rewarding and exciting road ahead. I suppose if I could give one main reason why I seriously became fascinated with anti-ageing and age-nostic medicine, it was the realization that I was in my mid-40s, divorced and alone. I had to rebuild my life, emotionally, physically and financially.

As you have seen from my chapter on addiction, my big problem has always been drinking too much at various times in my life. Not all the time, but when I seem to be getting too close to someone or at a difficult crossroads, I lapse back. I can tell you that the strategy of improvement through the consumption of large amounts of alcohol doesn't work and it is the worst thing you can do. It only brings on more depression and loneliness and unfortunately it has caused me to lose what could have been some good long-term relationships.

Second, at some point we have to get back on the horse and carry on in the right direction. Otherwise, it is easy to get into a downward spiral. I used alcohol to try to block everything out and all that happens is that the inevitable catches up with you. Usually after binges I was in a worse mental place for dealing with anything. I took up smoking heavily for a while, which was all linked. This is from someone who had already been living an age-nostic lifestyle for several years. The drink was making me self-harm.

While it's possible to recover fairly quickly when we are young, the body and mind take a lot longer as we grow older. This book has everything you will need to get back on top, and the amazing thing is that if you really don't give up, and really follow through, you will actually be in a better mental and physical shape than you had been 15 or 20 years earlier. I think that is one of the ironies of a massive change in life, such as divorce and taking the age-nostic approach; it is possible to come out feeling younger, happier and more positive than you ever thought you could be.

Second Time Around

This is a very controversial subject and one that can make many women quite angry. But I will write about it anyway because the book is written for men, so no apology here. The fact is that men second time around tend to go for younger women, but I think the reasons for this are often very misconstrued and not correct. You need to be youthful in your attitude towards life. You have to feel young and confident that you can get another partner; you won't have much chance if you are negative, overweight or in general bad shape. Assuming you are able to follow this book, you can have a great relationship with a younger woman, which can help to keep you younger. Alternatively, find someone with a similarly youthful mindset. I have a lot of younger friends, both male and female, and they bring a great deal to my life. I am not saying older people can't do this, but it is rare in my experience. The bottom line is to try to spend time with people who have a positive outlook and a desire to enjoy life to the full. For me, the energy and enthusiasm that younger women still have for life is the greatest attraction.

Recently, I was in Hotel de Paris in Monte Carlo. I was there to meet a potential partner in our pharmaceutical company, who has spent 15 years trying to find a way to work against the large companies and bring pharmaceutical supplements, with their great benefits, to market, which age-nostic medicine is based on. After dinner, we went to the hotel bar. The room was filled with men; many incredibly wealthy, others less so. Very few were under 40, most were over 50. If only I could talk to all of them and tell them about age-nostic medicine, I thought. When I do get to talk to such men, I always get a huge response. Maybe it is because we are not talking about money, success or material things. Instead we are talking about things which money cannot buy – health, youth, relationships and more time to enjoy life.

There were also some very beautiful women in the bar. Some were clearly escorts. Who am I to judge whether they want a handbag, house, baby or $2,000 for a night. I met a stunning Brazilian ex-model who I soon realized was a working girl. I told her I was not going to pay her for a night together. She was beautiful beyond belief but she was also intelligent, kind and full of energy, and we had a wonderful conversation. She was being genuine and not hiding what she needed: she had a four-year-old daughter to look after. On several occasions she left me to try to meet someone for the night, but having no luck, she eventually gave up and we talked for another three hours until the bar closed and she walked off into the night. It was just two people who enjoyed each other's company – me at 53, she at 29 – who didn't care in the end and were both a bit lonely.

Women are attracted to the energy, experience and confidence of men (especially those who are successful and who have power). But at the same time, men are energized by the attention and interest they receive from women (especially women younger than themselves). An obvious lesson for women is don't lose your energy and passion; if you do, you might lose your man. Men lose their energy and passion for life so easily, especially as they get older. Maybe that is why we seek it in younger partners, for it is never the sex; it is the energy in ourselves and our partners that we miss.

Ten tips for coping with relationships

1. Realize that all relationships are challenging.
2. You will have fewer close friends as you get older.
3. Keep as many young friends around you as possible.
4. Age in a great relationship is never a barrier.
5. See non-business friends as much as possible.
6. Don't get lonely and withdrawn.
7. Don't let age milestones mess with your head.
8. Don't stay because you think you are too old to leave.
9. Don't benchmark yourself against your peers.
10. Benchmark yourself with someone 10 to 15 years younger.

CHAPTER 12

A GENE NEAR YOU

The future of age-nostic
by Dr. Bob Goldman

Introduction by Dr. Michael Zacharia

I have had the unique opportunity of befriending Dr. Bob Goldman for more than 12 years now. He has regularly attended our Australian Anti-ageing Meeting, which is the little brother version of the outstanding A4M meeting. With his vast experience and expertise, I cannot think of anyone better than Bob to write this chapter on the future of age-nostic medicine.

By way of a short introduction, Dr. Robert M. Goldman M.D., Ph.D, DO, FAASP has spearheaded the development of numerous international medical organizations and corporations. Dr. Goldman authors the Anti-Ageing column published in the *Townsend Letter for Doctors & Patients*. In 2012, he was awarded the Life Time Achievement Award in Medicine & Science. Dr. Goldman is the recipient of the Gold Medal for Science, the Grand Prize for Medicine, the Humanitarian Award, and the Business Development Award. In addition, Dr. Goldman is a black belt in karate, Chinese weapons expert, world champion athlete with over 20 world strength records, and he has been listed in the Guinness Book of World Records. Some of his past performance records include 13,500 consecutive sit-ups and 321 consecutive handstand push-ups. Moreover, Dr. Goldman was awarded the Healthy American Fitness Leader Award from the President's Council on Physical Fitness & Sports and U.S. Chamber of Commerce.

The Future of Age-nostic Medicine
By Dr. Bob Goldman

I have been in the fortunate position of observing the progress in age rejuvenation techniques and technology and the future of age-nostic medicine is definitely here. Now! Only recently, the oldest woman to live was from Palestine who died aged 125 years in December 2012, and the oldest man recorded was 115 years old in January 2013. When I founded the American Academy of Anti-ageing Medicine (A4M) in 1993 with only 12 physicians, the oldest person recorded was approximately 110 years. Over the last 20 years, A4M has grown to over 26,000 global members from 120 nations, and at the same time we have seen an improvement in lifespan and importantly life quality as well. We know that getting older is inevitable, but ageing for the age-nostic man is optional, and it is for this reason I am happy to write about the future of age-nostic medicine in this book.

Age rejuvenation medicine focuses on the application of advanced scientific and medical technologies for the early detection, prevention, treatment and reversal of age-related dysfunction, disorders and diseases. It is a healthcare model that promotes innovative science and research to prolong the healthy lifespan in humans. The savings in disease-related costs of such an approach are clear. In the US alone, eliminating the number of deaths from cancer, heart disease, stroke, circulatory disease, influenza and AIDS would result in hundreds of billions of dollars returned to the economy (not including the savings in medical costs).

The elderly population in the US will double in size over the next 25 years as baby boomers reach retirement age. Eight in 10 Americans will be age 65 or over by year 2025. Today, boomers represent 28% of the US population and are the largest single sustained growth of the population in the history of the United States. Their mass alone has had an enormous impact on the national psyche, political arena and social fabric. By many measures, the baby boomer generation has redefined every life-cycle stage as they pass through it. In the 1960s and 1970s, they created a youth culture of rock n' rollers and hippies, who grew up to become the young urban professionals of the 1980s.

As a group, today's 50-somethings control 70% of the wealth in the US, own 77% of the financial assets, represent 66% of stockholders and own 80% of the money in savings accounts. As the oldest of the baby boomers approaches late adulthood, they are again poised to redefine the next stage in life – retirement. They are not willing to part with their tangible achievements of success prematurely: they seemingly universally yearn to retain their lean and mean mental and physical stature with each birthday, and they celebrate pushing anti-ageing health care to the forefront of clinical medicine. This is truly representative of the age-nostic man.

Anti-ageing medicine serves to fill a void in quality, wellness-oriented preventative healthcare that is sought specifically by baby boomers. Across the world they are seeking the medical expertise of anti-ageing physicians to provide very early detection, as well as aggressive yet gentle treatment of disease, to help them live long and fulfilling lives. A recent medical study suggests that 60% of people over the age of 65 are going outside the confines of disease-based medicine and seeking options to help them with enhancing their quality of life as they extend their quantity of life. As such, anti-ageing medicine does not prey on the ageing population; rather, this medical specialty protects the health and well-being of baby boomers and the elderly.

So, how are we going to get there? Any talk on the future of age-nostic medicine needs to consider what we know and have now, and how we can integrate future technologies to complement our current knowledge. As discussed in a recent presentation at the 2010 A4M Las Vegas meeting, Dr. Terry Grossman describes the future as a combination of three elements:

1. *Good health achieved by current medical practices, which includes a thorough history and examination, diagnosis and treatment, and prevention of disease processes.*

2. *The advancement of biotechnology.*

3. *The new age of nanotechnology.*

Good Health and Current Therapies

Caloric Restriction

Caloric restriction (CR) is a known intervention that might be able to delay human ageing. There is a large body of research on CR, especially with mice, and there are many products being developed to try to emulate its effects. It might be as simple as missing out on a few evening meals per week. However, we know that obesity and its consequences can shorten life dramatically and therefore the opposite may be true that caloric restriction may actually help to prolong life.

Hormonal Therapies

As we age, the levels of many hormones decrease. Some of the oldest and still most popular anti-ageing treatments are thus based on the notion that hormonal changes contribute to ageing and reversing age-related hormonal changes will be beneficial. The most famous of these treatments involves human growth hormone (HGH) injections. Growth hormone has a long history as an anti-ageing treatment and some evidence suggests HGH has beneficial effects in elderly people. HGH supplements might increase muscle mass, strengthen the immune system and increase libido. There are studies in elderly patients in which they claim to feel younger after HGH treatment. Some of the possible side effects of HGH include weight gain, high blood pressure and diabetes, but these are mostly reversible on removing the HGH or lowering its dose.

Other hormones whose production decreases with age include DHEA and melatonin. DHEA has been reported to improve the well-being of the elderly in a variety of ways: improved memory, immune system, muscle mass, sexual appetite and benefits to the skin. Protection against cancer has also been argued. Minor side effects such as acne have also been reported. Melatonin is a hormone mostly involved in sleep and circadian rhythms, the latter hypothesized by some to be associated with ageing and life extension. It appears to have antioxidant functions in the brain and may have some beneficial effects in elderly patients, in particular in terms of sleep. Some of its proponents claim it delays the ageing process and many age-related diseases. Although it can be used for jet lag and some sleep disorders, it may also cause sleep disorders such as nightmares and vivid dreams.

For women, oestrogen is a popular anti-ageing therapy. This hormone is generally used in conjunction with others in hormone replacement therapy. It does appear to reduce some of the effects of menopause by protecting against heart disease and osteoporosis. On the other hand, it could increase the risk of breast cancer and lead to weight gain and thrombosis as side effects. There is a vast literature on the advantages and disadvantages of hormone replacement therapy. For men, testosterone has also been touted as anti-ageing but, again, there is no evidence it has anti-ageing benefits even if it might have some benefits like, say, increased sexual function and muscle mass.

Antioxidants

One theory of ageing is the free radical theory. Succinctly, when oxygen is used to make energy in human cells, it releases reactive compounds called free radicals, also called reactive oxygen species (ROS). To fight ROS, cells possess an array of defences called antioxidants, many of which can be synthesized or extracted, purified and then sold, generally in tablets, as anti-ageing drugs. Common antioxidants include vitamins A, C and E and coenzyme Q10. Fortunately, there is probably little if nothing wrong with taking these products as serious side effects have not been described. Resveratrol, and other red wine constituents, can also act as antioxidants and might be protective agents of brain ageing. So antioxidants might be healthy in the same way vitamin supplements, often including antioxidants, may be healthy; on the other hand, one large study found no evidence that multivitamin use influences mortality. Since one major source of ROS is mitochondria, a similar class of compounds are aimed at quenching ROS production in mitochondria. These can include not only antioxidants, but products that allegedly "rejuvenate" mitochondria by optimizing metabolism or membrane potential. As with many other products, however, none of these products has been proven to have any effect on ageing, either in animal models or in humans.

Telomere-Based Therapies

Our cells are programmed to divide 30 to 50 times during the life span. Cells need to divide to repair tissue. Anything that causes cellular and/or tissue damage will lead to cellular division as the body attempts to repair the damage. Therefore, those 30 to 50 cell divisions get "used up" prematurely in the presence of damage caused by smoking, environmental toxins, poor nutrition and diseases like obesity, inflammatory diseases, cancer, heart disease and others. A major key to ageing well is keeping telomeres as long as possible. Optimal nutrition, regular exercise, optimal hormone levels and managing stress go a long way in preventing telomeres from getting too short "before their time". In addition, consumption of omega-3 fatty acids, vitamin D and other supplements can slow down telomere shortening.

Better yet, the first commercially available product tested in humans and shown to increase telomere length is now available. Its name is TA-65. TA-65 activates the enzyme telomerase, which repairs and restores telomere length. Telomerase is a naturally occurring enzyme in the body, but in our somatic cells (non-reproductive cells) is normally turned off. Studies of TA-65 in humans was shown to improve immune function, improve blood pressure, improve blood sugar and insulin levels, improve cholesterol profile and improve bone density. In addition, many study participants reported better energy, better sleep, better sexual performance and better visual acuity.

It's anticipated that even more potent telomerase activators will soon be available. So between stem cells and telomerase activators coupled with exercise, proper nutrition and hormonal optimization, the future looks bright and those who seek help from anti-ageing medicine will be able to live both a longer life and one of the highest quality.

Stem Cells

Stem cells have the ability to self-reproduce and differentiate into mature tissue like heart, liver and lung. Stem cell treatments have been and continue to be used to treat malignant and non-malignant blood-related diseases like leukaemia and lymphoma. Stem cells are also currently being used to treat heart failure, the leading cause of death in the United States. They are being studied in the treatment of a host of neurologic disorders like Parkinson's disease, stroke and spinal cord injury. Despite new treatments, complications from diabetes have not changed significantly and achieving glycemic control has been elusive. Emerging stem cell therapies to treat diabetes are showing promise as well.

In recent years, stem cells have received widespread attention. This fame is partly merited given the huge potential of stem cells for regenerative medicine. The possibility of using stem cells to treat diseases of ageing and for rejuvenation is also tantalizing. Harvesting and/or preparing stem cells for treatments is complex and much work remains to optimize protocols. In some areas, stem cells have been shown to be useful. For example, blood and marrow-derived stem cells have been used successfully in some autoimmune and cardiovascular diseases. Interestingly, mesenchymal stem cells transplanted from young donors did extend life span in mice. Yet stem cell applications are still in their infancy and there is a long way to go before physicians can employ stem cells to delay ageing.

ALT-711

ALT-711 is one of the latest anti-ageing compounds to receive public attention. It acts by catalytically breaking AGE crosslinks: Advanced Glycosylation End-product crosslinks occur when glucose is attached to a protein, as can happen in arteries. For this, ALT-711 seems to be useful against heart disease by reducing pulse pressure and improving arterial elasticity. The full effects and side effects of this drug are still unknown, but it seems like a promising intervention to ameliorate ageing's effects, though I remain sceptical – until proven contrary – that it can delay ageing as a whole.

Future Therapies

Rapamycin

One exciting finding in anti-ageing research was the discovery that feeding rapamycin, also known as sirolimus, to middle-aged mice extends lifespan by 9-14%. When fed to younger mice, rapamycin extends lifespan by 10-18%. Rapamycin is also an immunosuppressant, used to prevent organ rejection with serious side effects, and so it is not suitable as an anti-ageing drug. However, rapamycin works by inhibiting a complex pathway called TOR (Target of Rapamycin) and a number of labs and companies are now trying to target more specific downstream nodes of the pathway to develop anti-ageing drugs without the side effects of rapamycin.

Gene Therapy

Gene therapy is currently an experimental technique that uses genes to treat or prevent disease. At present, we can identify the human genome and specific disorders of the genome causing disease. In the near future, we will be able to treat a disorder by inserting a gene into a patient's cells instead of using drugs. Researchers are testing several approaches to gene therapy, including:

* *Deplacing a mutated gene that causes disease with a healthy copy of the gene.*
* *Inactivating or "knocking out" a mutated gene that is functioning improperly.*
* *Introducing a new gene into the body to help fight a disease.*

One gene that appears to influence ageing in mice is klotho. High levels of klotho increase lifespan by about 30%, though it is not entirely clear if ageing is delayed and low levels appear to foster ageing. Human longevity has also been linked to allelic variants in this gene. Its functions are still largely a mystery, but since the gene encodes one secreted form that acts as a hormone, it could be synthesized and presented as an anti-ageing therapy. For now, however, we will just have to wait and see. There are many other ageing-associated genes that hold promise for pharmaceutical intervention, and progress has been made in finding chemicals that can modulate specific ageing-associated genes and thus extend lifespan.

Biotechnology and Nanomedicine

A nanometre is one billionth of a metre or 0.7 of the width of a human hair. Nanomedicine looks at using medications or robots embedded in the nanometre size to invade small spaces and target specific parts of the body. The combination of biotechnology with nanomedicine will provide exciting changes in scientific and economic development. The European Science Foundation defines nanomedicine as "the science and technology of diagnosing, treating and preventing disease and traumatic injury, of relieving pain, and of preserving and improving human health, using molecular tools and molecular knowledge of the human body". In the very near future, we will be able to develop new techniques for characterizing the internal structures of cells and duplicate the properties of the molecular machines found in living systems.

Among its many emerging benefits, nanomedicine may facilitate the oral administration of drugs that are currently delivered only by injection.

Nanoencapsulation of such drugs in a minuscule polymer or lipid matrix will allow them to easily pass through the gastrointestinal lining and reach the bloodstream where their payload will be released. Additionally, nanoparticles, which can be as small as a virus, can efficiently enter into diseased cells and facilitate more effective diagnosis and treatment. In whichever application, nanomedicine will drastically improve a patient's quality of life by early detection and/or more efficient treatment with less drug-related side effects. Overall, expansion of these nanopharmaceuticals will improve the practice of medicine and clinical outcomes in the coming years.

Nanorobots might be able to seek out cancer cells and kill them without affecting other normal cells, which is what chemotherapy does; nanoparticles can attach drugs to them that might be able to enter individual cells and deliver their treatment directly in high concentrations or carry antibodies to a cell or chemotherapeutic agents directly into cells.

In Conclusion

Even though there is not a single magic pill at present that will retard ageing, there are simple lifestyle and dietary adjustments that can make you live longer. Most components of a healthy lifestyle are well known already. A varied, rich diet with plenty of fruits and vegetables that is low in carbohydrates and fat is likely to make you live longer. As an example, look at the Okinawan population in Japan, where older individuals have a lower risk of age-related chronic diseases and mortality when compared to the rest of Japan. Okinawans tend to avoid high calorie sugars, saturated fats and processed foods and instead consume more vegetables and fruits, which is likely to contribute to their longer life. Conversely, smoking, excess alcohol, obesity, lack of exercise and high blood pressure are all associated with higher mortality. One study showed that middle-aged (45-64 years of age) people who adopted a healthy lifestyle by consuming five or more fruits and vegetables daily, regular exercise, healthy body mass index (BMI) (18.5-29.9 kg/m2) and not smoking experienced a prompt benefit in lower rates of cardiovascular disease and mortality. Clearly, not smoking, exercise, moderate alcohol intake and fruit and vegetable intake are associated with lower mortality. Again, we know that getting older is inevitable, but ageing for the age-nostic man is optional.

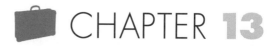

CHAPTER 13

THE JOURNEY
CONTINUES

What does an age-nostic future hold for me?

I don't find this an easy question to answer. What I have learned over the last 10 years has given me tremendous quality of life because my body has felt younger. One thing I have gleaned from this journey is that life is very precious and many of us do tend to take it for granted in our younger years. We abuse our bodies when we are seemingly invincible, only to suffer the consequences when we get older. I also feel that too many of us think it is too late to change.

I have learned enough in the past decade or so to know that a revolution in the ageing process is happening right now. Once the knowledge is refined and made accessible to all men, we will all benefit from it if we are brave enough and not concerned about change. The medical fraternity and many in society are highly suspicious of anything to do with anti-ageing, and I can only imagine what criticism this book is going to get when it is published. I am happy to take the flak it will generate because someone needs to be controversial in this space.

The next 20 years or so for me are going to be the most exciting and rewarding of my life as I continue to learn more, experiment more and live a happier, healthier and younger life. I truly believe that science is about to make the most incredible breakthroughs in medicine and profoundly affect the ageing process as we understand it; much of which we can't even begin to comprehend at this point. It has been the same in medicine for centuries.

I love going to anti-ageing conferences and hearing that humans, in the not-too-distant future, could be living to an age of 120, 140 or even 160 years. I mention this to people and many respond by saying, "Who wants to live to 150 years?" This is because the perception of the quality of life at that age is so poor. We have all seen old people who can hardly walk or get around. However, with the developments in anti-ageing medicine, things don't have to be like that. We can still be mentally alert and physically able to do a great deal. Wouldn't it be a fantastic achievement to run a marathon on my 100th birthday?

There is a certain satisfaction in reaching the age of 50 and still feeling like a 30-year-old. Hopefully you are now a bit more informed about what is available and therefore will find it easier to explore a few new paths. I will continue to hunt out any new treatments and solutions to keep on top of the medical developments. I will continue to research anti-ageing and try to live every day as if I am still 30 years old. I truly believe that by following my regime and continuing to experiment with new breakthroughs, anyone can age more slowly and improve their quality of life.

The Anti-ageing Business

From a business and career perspective, I am excited about being able to bring a great deal of what I have learned to others. I have pulled together a group of real experts in this field and after much research and planning, we have created a company called Genagenostic.com. Our mission is to create a series of clinics throughout the world that will give every man access to the best anti-ageing treatments and advice. The business will also be a platform for new discoveries and thinking. We will continue to focus on the three pillars of age-nostic medicine (mood, energy and vitality) and after the opening of our first clinic in Los Angeles in late 2013, we will be producing our own range of specially designed gen-agenostic supplements. We will then open clinics in several other major cities around the world.

We have also gone into a joint venture with an exclusive resort group to provide retreats to give men access to intensive life-transforming programmes. This will fast-track the age-nostic journey and get participants on a new path as quickly as possible. I am simply more excited about the future and in better physical and spiritual shape than I ever was in my 30s. I am also more productive than I have ever been in my life. To me, this feels like a great gift and something I believe in with a passion. I don't want to change the world, but if just one man can feel the way I do and roll back the years, then I will be content that I chose to write this book.

One of the best parts of this whole journey to date has been the people

I have met and talked to about anti-ageing and the age-nostic approach. While admittedly there was some scepticism at the start, they have become convinced that real change is possible. Each of them has made some personal discoveries that have led to a change in their own ageing process. We are just a group of ageing blokes who want nothing more than to feel great and enjoy the remaining years. From a personal point of view, I am particularly interested in stem cell treatment and I am already undergoing various treatments using my own stem cells. The initial results I have been getting are excellent, and hopefully I will get a chance to write another book to reveal all the fantastic opportunities stem cells can bring to all of us.

Breaking New Ground

For sure, most of what has been written in this book has never been assembled in one book before. I was most reluctant to put down many of my own personal experiences, failures and falls from grace, but it has been a helpful process. In the past, I was much more interested in discussing my successes, but now they seem less exciting. I have tried to look at the whole process of growing older and not just the glossy or easy-to-discuss parts. Through revealing my own experiences and those of the other contributors, we hope you will be able to relate more to the solutions we recommend. We have all been excited by what we have experienced and found out about ourselves in this continuous journey of falling, getting up, falling and getting up again.

There are thousands of motivational books, health programmes, diets, etc. on the market today and the vast majority just don't work for normal people. They are not real enough and not holistic enough to make a difference. What is the point of losing weight if you still have a problem with addiction or depression? What is the point of starting a new exercise programme if you still drink and eat too much? Elements of our lives can't be disconnected, and we must look at everything that affects the health of our body and mind. I believe the key points of this book are two-fold:

1. You can completely reverse the ageing process in a dramatic way.

2. If you don't act, the journey is pretty well laid out and for most people the picture doesn't look that good.

We all make choices in life. The hard thing is to live with them and accept them. In my life, I have made some huge mistakes, but I am very lucky to not have the regret gene and that is one of the greatest gifts a man can have when he starts getting older. If you do have that, look at ways to lessen the impact on your outlook and behaviour. It is no coincidence that as a man reaches middle age, he begins to look back on his life and starts regretting things. Did he choose the right partner? Did he choose the right career? Did he look after himself when he had energy and youth?

And then he reaches his 40s and it all comes into sight. Maybe this is what the mid-life crisis is actually all about. Perhaps it is not a physical experience alone, but a simple feeling that many things we wanted to achieve may have passed us by.

We all remember from our childhood what it was like to miss out on something: not get invited to the birthday party; not make the sports team; not attract the girl we thought we loved. We went through the pain of loss and then found quickly that there were many more great things to look forward to. In all these experiences, we always had the future ahead of us. We always had our health, both mental and physical, which helped get us through any crisis, and we could quickly recover. Then it would be onto the next adventure, the next experience, the next job or the next love affair.

We could get fired from a job and go to the pub the same evening with friends as if nothing had happened. We had the energy and hope that all would be alright because we had time on our side. We could smoke and drink when we wanted and never worry about the consequences.

Public Interest in Anti-ageing

It never ceases to amaze me the amount of interest I get when I talk to people about age-nostic medicine. There are always two natural responses, suspicion and reluctance, especially from those who have already prematurely aged. However, in every case to date when I talked about my own experiences, my own journey and results, there was always excitement and enthusiasm. It often led to the question, "So where do I get it?" I am also surprised at how many men in their late 20s show so much enthusiasm for age-nostic medicine. I believe it shows that even at that age, many are worried about their own ageing process.

If I had to come up with one statement that sums up this book and the age-nostic man, it would be the following:

It's all out there if you are brave and passionate enough to access it. You have seen the alternative way to age and it just may be that this is a better way.

This is because the only retirement the age-nostic man should ever think about is death, and you don't need any cash in your grave. You need to fight the process of ageing mentally as much as physically, and it is a battle worth fighting because the life you can lead for many years can be much more exciting, healthy and happy.

I am an extreme case, and I am an extreme person, and have experimented with most things. I will continue because I am enjoying life in my 50s. I believe 50s are the new 30s. Some people ask me about my long-term health after they have read something on the Internet that scared them about hormone replacement, new anti-ageing drugs or supplements. I find it amusing in a way because things have been so positive for so many people. I have seen the long-term effects of the present ageing process all over the world and would much prefer to live my life the age-nostic way than to continue on the traditional path.

Enjoy your journey and just be yourself, because everyone else is taken.

Appendix 1
Contributor Biographies

Dr. Michael Zacharia

Dr. Michael Zacharia is a practicing ENT/Facial Plastic Surgeon who also has had a long interest in anti-ageing medicine. He is past Chairman of the Younger Fellows Committee for the Royal Australasian College of Surgeons along with Past President of the Australasian College of Cosmetic Surgery (ACCS), Past President of The Australasian Academy of Anti-ageing Medicine (A5M) and Treasurer of The Australasian Academy of Facial Plastic Surgery (AAFPS). He continues to be active with both educational bodies in the role of teaching and examination of trainees, administration and lecturing at their annual conferences. Dr. Zacharia also lectures internationally at cosmetic and anti-ageing conferences including A4M, IMCAS, ECAAM and AAFPRS.

Tim Watson-Munro

Tim Watson-Munro is a forensic psychologist, academic and author. He has assessed in excess of 20,000 clients and appeared in court as an expert witness over 3,000 times. He is a former Visiting Fellow at Melbourne University and Adjunct Visiting Professor at Bond University and has sat on various Advisory Boards with these institutions. Tim is regularly featured in the media, including being the former Resident Psychologist on Radio 3AW Drive Time, a columnist for the *Herald Sun*, and an expert commentator on aspects of forensic profiling and psychology for *Time* magazine and the BBC.

Phil Micans

Phil Micans, MS, PharmB, is an author, lecturer, editor and anti-ageing veteran. He studied Food & Vitamin Technology at South London College and afterwards he completed an Applied Science Bachelor's Degree in Pharmacy. He also holds a Masters Degree in Biochemistry from the University of Canterbury. Having been actively involved in the anti-ageing field since the 1980s, Phil has held the positions of Editor-in-Chief of the *Ageing Matters™ Magazine*, Director of Research and Development to *IM Health*, co-writer of *The New Millennium Guide to Anti-ageing Medicine* and Chairman of the Monte Carlo Anti-ageing Congress and is currently Assistant Editor to the *Lifespan Medicine Magazine™*. Phil realized that the information age has created a new generation of informed individuals and physicians who view things globally and want to obtain the best possible treatment based on a scientific perspective. As such, in 1991 he became a founding member of *International Anti-ageing Systems* (IAS), where he maintains the position of Vice President.

Appendix 2
Further Reading to Enhance your Healthcare Programme

Passion, sex and longevity, the oxytocin adventure
Thierry Hertoghe, M.D.
If you want to learn all about oxytocin, the so-called love hormone, then this is the book. It describes exactly what oxytocin is, how it has been used and all the uses it has been put to. Dr. Hertoghe is one of Europe's leading endocrinologists and his unique practical style provides a real "how-to" guide to oxytocin.

Stay 40 without diet and exercise
Richard Lippman, Ph.D.
Dr. Lippman has been nominated for the Nobel Prize in medicine for his work in free radicals. In this book, Dr. Lippman describes the right way to use potent free radical scavengers to protect yourself from ageing. In addition, he describes the interaction of supplementing certain hormones and other unique beneficial agents to delay and reverse all aspects of ageing.

Maximize your vitality and potency
Jonathan Wright, M.D.
Dr. Wright is one of America's leading endocrinologists and in this book he describes exactly how men can protect themselves from the "male menopause". He details the responsible ways of improving testosterone levels to ensure protection against flab, depression and sexual deterioration for men.

Smart drugs II - the next generation
Ward Dean, M.D.
Dr. Dean's book describes how various medicines and specialist nutrients can be used by people to protect them against age-related mental decline.

If memory loss is a concern for you or if your job requires considerable cognition, alertness or concentration, then with this book you can learn how you can improve all of those functions.

The key of life
Walter Pierpaoli, M.D.

Dr. Pierpaoli's book updates his best-seller *The Melatonin Miracle*. Discover how and why this single hormone operates. It is not only a godsend for jet lag and shift-work, it also enhances your immune system, thus enabling the correct hormonal responses each day. Learn how that in turn protects against serious conditions and enhances one's joy of life.

Grow young with HGH
Ronald Klatz, M.D.

Dr. Klatz highlights the research behind the anti-ageing hormone GH or growth hormone. GH is not just the domain of body builders to build muscle and lose fat; it has other significant clinically proven properties such as improving skin thickness and elasticity, improving hair condition, as well as enhancing well-being and outlook on life. If you are interested in GH, this is the book to have.

Better sex through chemistry
John Morgenthaler

This book does exactly what it says on the cover! It details how all kinds of different agents have been shown to affect and enhance sexual performance. From the desire to have sex (libido) to issues of erectile dysfunction to improving aspects of love-making itself, this book has it all.

Vitamin C, infectious diseases and toxins, curing the incurable
Thomas Levy, M.D.

Everything you ever needed to know about the power of vitamin C is here. Not only does Dr. Levy include a mass of well-structured information about the enormous scope of the benefits of vitamin C, the book also includes all the published references – so your doctor can't deny it!

Testosterone for life

Abraham Morgenthaler, M.D.

Written by an expert in testosterone therapy, this book covers all aspects of testosterone and testosterone supplementation in a witty and accessible style. Drawing on 30 years' research, the author discusses the role of this hormone in the body, symptoms of its deficiency, safe supplementation and its benefits, plus the latest scientific breakthroughs.

About the Author

Michael Hogg is a serial entrepreneur with a global track record of success across a number of industries.

More recently he was the global CEO of The Cobra Group of Companies. Over the last decade Michael was instrumental in driving a change agenda, which lead to a significant growth phase for the Group worldwide. He also masterminded Cobra's initial series of investments into a number of highly successful publicly listed enterprises.

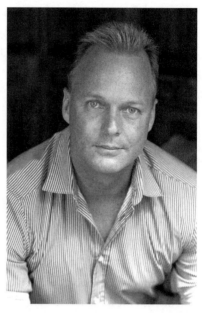

Having achieved everything he set out to achieve as a CEO, Michael decided to pursue his passion in anti-ageing. For over 10 years, Michael has been researching and experimenting in anti-ageing for men – the result being a biological age of 53 but a medical age of 30 to 35.

This has lead to Michael incubating the Gen-a business, which is dedicated to raising awareness and providing education to a new generation of men, and to enable them to access a range of age-nostic treatments. This new generation of men will be positioned to achieve the amazing results Michael has achieved on his own age-nostic journey.

This book is for...

Romy and Asha who accepted their mad crazy Dad with love. Paul for believing and being such an amazing friend. Boudou who kept my finger on the keyboard when I couldn't write. For Sasha who was there at the start. Rosie who was there for the longest and the worst times. Michael Abboud for his passion and courage to jump on board. To Isabella who just told me to breath and got me to the finish.

Acknowledgements

To the boys at Home House London, Andrew, Ian, Reece and Joel, who gave me a home to write in when I was in London. To Chris who believed in me and backed me as usual. To Paul and Richard who were there as normal all these years.

To Sara for a wonderful cover and all the staff at Singapore Airlines who looked after me so well on those long flights and to whomever sat next to me and let me work all night with the light on. And of course to Tim, Michael, Phil and Jonathon who wrote their parts on a handshake.

BEYOND
THE WRITTEN WORD

Authors who speak to you face to face.

Discover LID Speakers, a service
that enables businesses to have
direct and interactive contact with
the best ideas brought to their
own sector by the most
outstanding creators
of business thinking.

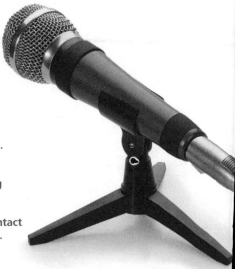

- A network specialising in business
  speakers, making it easy to find the
  most suitable candidates.

- A website with full details and videos,
  so you know exactly who you're hiring.

- A forum packed with ideas and
  suggestions about the most interesting
  and cutting-edge issues.

- A place where you can make direct contact
  with the best in international speakers.

- The only speakers' bureau backed up
  by the expertise of an established
  business book publisher.

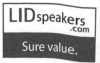